Journey
—to a—
Non-Toxic
Home

The Room-by-Room Guide to a Natural, Healthy Home

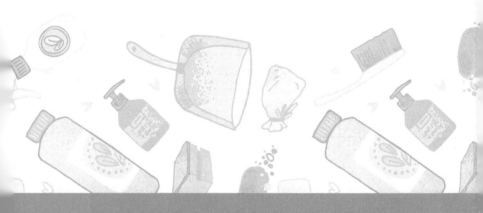

SARAH UMMYUSUF

Copyright © 2021 by Sarah UmmYusuf

All rights reserved. No part of this publication may be reproduced or transmitted in any form or by any means, electronic or mechanical, including photocopying, recording, or any other information storage and retrieval system, without the written permission of the publisher.

First paperback edition January 2021

Edited by Cindy Dockendorff
Proofread by Susan Sparke
Design and layout by Ljiljana Pavkov
Cover design by Stojan Mihajlov

ISBN 978-1-7775154-0-9 (paperback)
ISBN 978-1-7775154-1-6 (ebook)

Published by Nurtured Life Publishing
c/o Nature's Nurture
www.naturesnurtureblog.com

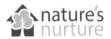

Disclaimer: The information made available in this book is for informational and educational purposes only. This information has not been evaluated by the Food and Drug Administration, and is not intended to diagnose, treat, cure, or prevent any disease. The author is not liable for the misuse of the information provided in this book.

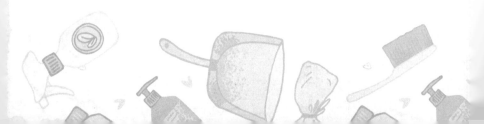

For my husband and children

Thank you for believing in my dream.
No work is more important than my love for you.

P.S. I can come to the park with you now. ♥

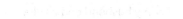

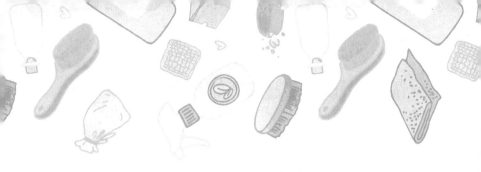

Contents

Journey

— to a —

Non-Toxic

Home

"

Don't forget—no one else sees
the world the way you do, so no
one else can tell the stories that
you have to tell.

— CHARLES DE LINT

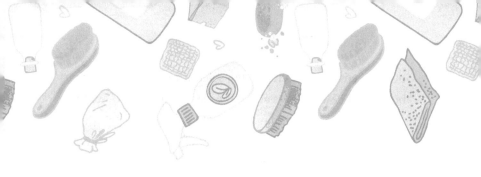

AUTHOR'S NOTE

Many people don't know this, but I was initially very reluctant to write this book. I probably shouldn't be telling you that, but it's the truth. I thought everything I wanted to say was already out there in the hundreds of other books written on this topic, and I couldn't imagine what new contributions I could bring to an already saturated market.

But then I had a moment of clarity while speaking with a close friend, and she helped me realize that it's not about inventing something new. It's about presenting the information differently, from a different point of view. And that's when it dawned on me that I've already been doing that through my online presence for nearly a decade.

My blog, Nature's Nurture, began as a side hobby that I indulged as a new mom during those long, sleepless nights, and in between diaper changes and nap times. Today, it's a thriving community of ordinary people trying to do the extraordinary: protect their families from harmful chemicals. Through my work over these last 10 years, I've pored over dozens of research articles, scientific studies, and various books and news articles about the use—and overuse—of toxic chemicals in our everyday household products.

I finally decided to write this book because I wanted to create the very thing I wish I'd had when I began my non-toxic journey. I needed a dynamic guide instead of an oversimplified to-do list. Someone to hold my hand and mentor me instead of making me feel like I was never going to get this right. I needed something personal, approachable, and easy to digest instead of a textbook filled with random facts that I couldn't easily apply to my life.

That's what this book is: a personal guide that's easy to understand and implement. This book will meet you where you are on your journey, and not in some arbitrary place where you "should" be.

It is more than just another green cleaning recipe book—although you'll find plenty of those in here, too! Because while 100+ recipes crammed into a small book would for sure be a useful resource, recipes are just one small piece of a much larger puzzle. I want to help you understand the *why* of this journey before we get into the *what* and the *how*.

So, this is your official invitation. Join me as we dive deep into the world of natural living and let me show you how you too can start your journey to a non-toxic home.

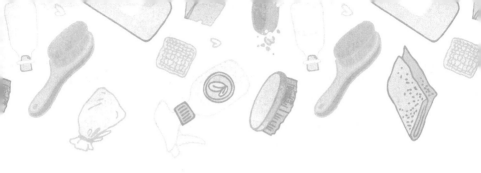

INTRODUCTION

everal years ago, when my oldest child, Yusuf, was a wee toddler, I went through one of the most terrifying experiences any young mother could imagine. The memory haunts me to this day, and it took me a very long time to get over the ensuing "mom guilt" that followed.

It was a day just like any other; I was home with Yusuf. He was playing in the kitchen as I worked quickly to prepare dinner. And then it happened. I went to the bathroom, and not even two minutes after I left, I heard screaming coming from the kitchen. I rushed back to the kitchen, completely unprepared for what I saw.

The cabinet under the kitchen sink was wide open, and there was Yusuf huddled inside, crying, screaming, and frantic.

But from what? What did he get into? And why was he in so much pain?

When I got a closer look, I could see a white, chalky powder all over his mouth and hands, dribbling down his chin and onto his shirt. Scared and confused, I looked around to try

3

to picture what could have happened in the two minutes that I was gone—and then I saw it. A large plastic tub of dishwasher detergent pods. He had managed to pry open the cover, take one out, and bite right into it, in true toddler fashion.

I freaked out. I panicked. I froze. I was not prepared for anything like this, and all I could think was, *oh my God, what have I done?!*

Long story short, he was completely fine, thankfully. After I washed his face and mouth, I called poison control. They told me what to do, what to look for, and how to handle the next couple of hours. But there was something else the poison control professional told me that shook me to my core: "This kind of thing happens all the time."

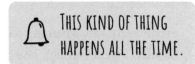

THIS KIND OF THING HAPPENS ALL THE TIME.

Yusuf was lucky. He got off with some minor discomfort and was back to his old self in no time. But too many children (and pets) are hospitalized every year for this exact thing! I'm grateful that my son was spared, but I couldn't shake the thought of how much worse it could have been.

And the irony of this whole thing?

That tub of detergent pods wasn't even ours! We had just moved into a new home, and it was left behind by the previous tenants. But it could very well have been ours, and that was all I needed. That experience lit a fire under me, and it's what got me seriously into this non-toxic lifestyle.

Let's rewind to a few months before Yusuf was born, to 2011, when I started my blog, Nature's Nurture. I was trying recipes for a few homemade products, and some friends and family asked me to share those recipes with them.

Instead of emailing them the same word document over and over again, I asked my techie husband to help me set up a little website where I could share whatever I wanted.

And that's all I had ever envisioned for my blog—just a place in my tiny corner of the internet to share recipes with people I know.

But life has a way of surprising you and exceeding even your wildest expectations.

I truly believe that fearful day with Yusuf was a sign from God. A sign that I needed to do more. That I needed to learn more, share more, and be more. For my family, yes, but also for the hundreds and thousands of women just like me who were looking for a better way to protect themselves and their families from harmful chemicals.

So in 2012, barely one week after the detergent incident, I decided to go full force with Nature's Nurture and grow it into what it is today: a place to learn, grow, and thrive on your journey to a non-toxic home. A place to find the confidence and peace of mind you need to protect your family from harmful chemicals. A place to help you finally take charge of your family's health and well-being.

And that's why I wrote this book.

Through years of blogging about my own journey, and then mentoring and coaching families through theirs, I've learned a few things, and I wanted to put them all in one place.

The book you're holding in your hands has truly been a labour of love. I pray that it benefits you and gives you just what you need to confidently and faithfully embark on your journey to a non-toxic home.

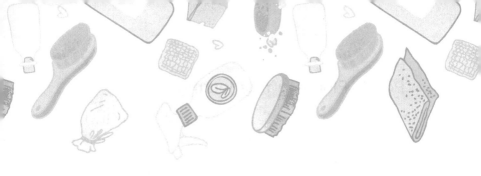

How to Use This Book

This book is divided into four parts, each with its own set of goals to get you one step closer to your non-toxic home. To help illustrate these different parts, let's use a simple analogy of building a house from the ground up.

Part I: The Truth About Household Products

This is the foundation of the book. It's the strong base that holds up your home and gives it lasting stability for years to come. This is where you'll find the research and knowledge that will set you up with everything you need to move forward on your journey.

Be warned: it's also the section that will frustrate you the most. We'll look at how common household products can affect our health. We'll learn about how our governments test and regulate the chemicals we are exposed to every day. We'll also explore some of the most harmful chemicals in our products, and how to limit our exposure to them.

Part II: Planning Your Journey

This is the structure of the book. It's the solid frame that holds up the walls and roof, protecting your home from buckling under the force of strong winds and storms.

I'll help you get clear on your goals, come up with your Why Statement, and take your very first step to a non-toxic home. This is where I share the roadmap and formula you'll use throughout your journey. And if you're worried about family members sabotaging your efforts, there's also a special chapter here just for you.

Part III: The Room-by-Room Analysis

This part is what we could call the furnishings. Here we find the functional and beautiful pieces that will adorn your home, giving it a cozy and comfortable atmosphere. This is where you'll take everything you've learned so far and put it into action in the room-by-room walkthrough—my absolute favourite part!

I'm going to take you on a virtual tour of your entire home and show you exactly what to look for and where to focus your efforts for maximum results. I'll give you simple options for finding and using safer alternatives to the products you're currently using. Just imagine that you've invited me over for coffee, and we'll casually stroll through your home, moving from room to room as we discuss how we're going to help you achieve your goals for a natural, healthy home.

Part IV: Looking Ahead

This final part will wrap it all up for you and give you concrete steps that you can take to start your journey as soon as you finish the book. I'll give you a quick recap of everything we've learned, an Action Plan that you can customize for your family, and a Quick Start Guide with some of the easiest products you can switch out right away.

We'll end it off with a little pep talk for encouragement, because who doesn't love a nice pat on the back to get you on your way?

Remember: Build from the Ground Up

I strongly encourage you to begin with Part I and read this book in the order that it's laid out. Don't just skip through to the final section, looking for the recipes and product recommendations. You wouldn't start furnishing your home until you've laid the foundation and secured the frame in place, right?

I know it's tempting to dive right in, but I promise you'll be better off if you embark on this journey by working your way from the ground up.

Website Links

Please note that there are a lot of website links in this book. You can type them directly into your web browser to access them at any time. To make it easier for you, I have also created a special page on my website that includes all the links, resources, and references mentioned in this book. To access the page simply go to: naturesnurtureblog.com/book

Are you ready? Let's jump right into Part I and learn the truth about common household products and how they can affect our health.

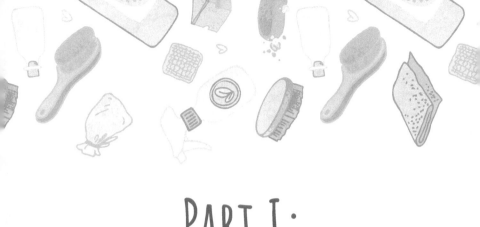

Part I:

The Truth About Household Products

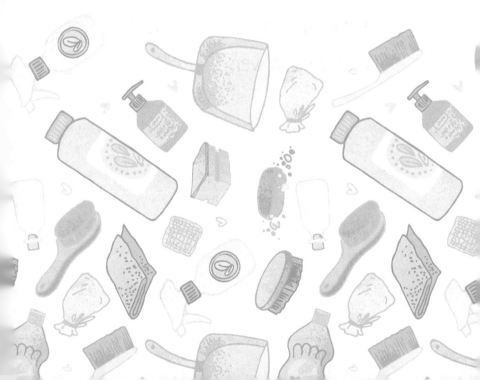

"

If we are going to live so
intimately with these chemicals
eating and drinking them, taking
them into the very marrow of
our bones—we had better know
something about their nature
and their power.

— RACHEL CARSON, *SILENT SPRING*

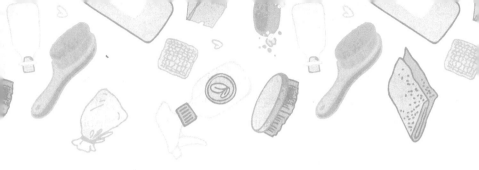

CHAPTER 1:

CAN OUR CLEANING PRODUCTS MAKE US SICK?

One day many years ago, after moving into a new rental home, I opened the shower stall in the master bathroom and was met with an unsightly amount of dark mould all along the grout lines. It was everywhere—the floor, the walls, the corners, and all the crevices in between.

It was horrible. And I was at a complete loss because I had no idea how to remove it without resorting to harsh, toxic chemicals. After all, what's the first thing you're taught to reach for if you want to get rid of mould in a bathroom? Bleach. But as we'll learn in Chapter 5, household bleach comes with its own list of health risks and side effects. And I didn't want to risk it.

So I closed the shower stall, walked away, and decided to just use one of the other showers in the house for the duration of our lease. Of course, this only lasted for so long before I finally gave in and resolved to tackle this mould situation once and for all—even if it meant having to use a little bleach to get the job done.

That same day, I went out—dragging my feet the whole way—and bought a mainstream mould and mildew spray. I prepared myself as much as possible to try to mitigate the effects of the harsh chemicals I was about to spray all over my tiny shower stall; I ran the exhaust fan, I opened the bathroom window—in the middle of February in Canada! I put on some rubber gloves and wrapped a scarf around my face so I wouldn't have to inhale the fumes directly.

And as I stood there in my bathroom, dressed in my makeshift HAZMAT suit, mentally preparing myself for the assault I was about to unleash on all my senses, I felt an overwhelming sense of sadness and frustration.

Sadness, because I know millions of people use these harsh products in their homes without even thinking about it, let alone protecting themselves as I had. And frustration, because I couldn't understand how and why products like this are allowed to be sold on shelves under the guise of "generally regarded as safe."

Safe for whom, exactly? Was this product tested in a controlled environment? Did the manufacturer have to prove that this product wouldn't cause long-term health problems? Was each individual ingredient in this product analyzed and put through a rigorous evaluation before it was released?

So many questions scrambled through my mind in those few seconds, but I knew the answer to all of them. It was a loud and resounding *NO*. The products we use to clean and freshen our homes are not tested, analyzed, or evaluated before hitting the market—at least not in the way we expect them to be, but I'll talk more about this in the next chapter.

I eventually did clean that shower stall. It was rough and I had to take a few breaks along the way, but I got through it. And although the spray helped remove the mould, it didn't get rid of all of it. And you know what that means—I was supposed to keep using it regularly for "maintenance." But I couldn't bring myself to use it ever again.

Household Chemicals and Our Health

Our health starts on the inside. We hear this repeatedly from medical professionals, nutritionists, personal trainers, and anyone in the health and wellness industry. We know it's important to eat a nutritious diet and get regular exercise if our goal is to live a happy, healthy life.

But let me take it one step further and say that's not where our health stops. What we put *on* and *around* our bodies is just as important as what we put *in* them. If your diet is on track and you're moving your body regularly, but your household and personal care products contain harmful toxins unfortunately, you're missing a major piece of the puzzle.

Volatile Organic Compounds (VOCs)

Here's the thing: the products you use in your home don't stay locked away in your cabinet all day. Each time you take one out and clean your counter with it, spray it in the air, or scrub your floor with it, it's releasing tiny chemicals called *volatile organic compounds* into the air you breathe.

15

Volatile organic compounds (VOCs) are a large group of chemicals that exist in both indoor and outdoor air. They are released into indoor air from many sources, including furniture, building materials, fragrance products, plastics, and cleaning products, to name a few.

VOCs and Our Health

Short-term exposure to high levels of VOCs can cause breathing problems and headaches, as well as irritation of the eyes, nose, and throat. People with asthma can be especially sensitive to these compounds.[1]

On the other hand, **long-term** exposure to high levels of VOCs (for example, in industrial workers) has been linked to increased cancer rates[2] and damage to the liver and kidneys.[3]

But most of us don't fall into either of those categories. For the average family home, we're dealing with lower levels of VOCs over a long period of time. Right now, research is still ongoing to study the long-term effects of the lower levels that are typically found in homes. But one thing is for sure: these chemicals are no good and we should be reducing our exposure to them as much as possible.

VOCs and Indoor Air Pollution

Did you know that the Environmental Protection Agency (EPA) considers poor indoor air quality to be "among the top five environmental risks to public health"?[4] Yes, you read that right—the air inside our homes, schools, and offices is a top public health risk!

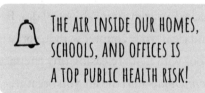

THE AIR INSIDE OUR HOMES, SCHOOLS, AND OFFICES IS A TOP PUBLIC HEALTH RISK!

A 2016 Canadian study comparing indoor/outdoor air quality ratios found indoor concentrations of VOCs to be higher than the outdoor air in all but one of the 25 VOCs that were studied.[5] Isn't that just wild? When I think of pollution, I think of smog, car exhaust, and trash littering the streets and waterways. I never once considered that my own home could be a source of pollution—and a significant one, at that.

Four simple ways to improve indoor air quality

1. Bring plants into your indoor spaces. Chapter 14 has a section on Air Purifying Houseplants and how they remove (or reduce) VOCs from the air.
2. Leave your shoes at the door. Don't track all of that dirt, bacteria, and toxins into your home.
3. Dust regularly to remove particles that can aggravate or induce mild allergies.
4. Open the windows to air out your space on a regular basis—even (and especially) in the winter.

Now look, if you're only exposed to a tiny amount of these chemicals a few times in your life, they probably won't cause any harm. But with repeated exposure over a long period—and in combination with the hundreds of other chemicals you're exposed to in any given week—they can build up in your body and eventually lead to chronic disease.

But how, exactly, does this happen? To answer this question, we first have to understand exactly how our bodies process these chemicals.

The Burden on Our Bodies

I recently learned that our bodies begin accumulating toxins and pollutants on the day we are born. That's right; since your very first day on this big, green Earth, your body has been collecting and storing tiny bits of chemicals in your bones, your blood, your body fat, and even in breastmilk.[6]

The total number of toxins in our bodies at any given time is known as the **total body burden**. From the air we breathe to the food we eat, to the water we drink and bathe in, we're constantly being exposed to various toxins in the environment, whether we're aware of it or not. These toxins can be anything from dangerous heavy metals to pesticides on our food, and yes, even the chemicals in our household products.

The good news is that our body has mechanisms in place—namely, the liver and kidneys—to process and flush these toxins out of our systems. The bad news? When our bodies are exposed to more toxins than it can handle, the liver and kidneys become overloaded and are unable to function properly.

Toxic overload can be a heavy burden on the body. Depending on several factors, including how much, for how long, and how often someone is exposed, chemicals can have different effects on different people. And when toxins aren't processed and eliminated from the body properly, they can build up in fatty tissue and organs, putting your body and overall health under greater stress.

REMEMBER:

While it's important to look at your diet and exercise, it's equally important to examine the chemicals that you allow into your immediate environment and how they can affect your health and well-being. Because although our health starts on the inside, that's not where it stops.

In the next chapter, we're going to learn about what makes conventional household products so sneaky, and why cleaning product companies are allowed to get away with it.

"

The truth will set you free,
but first it will piss you off.

—Joe Klaas, *The Twelve Steps to Happiness*

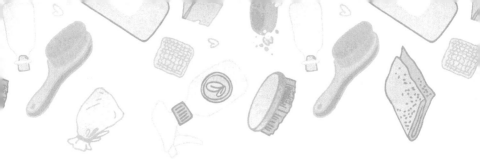

CHAPTER 2:
WHAT IS HIDING IN OUR HOUSEHOLD PRODUCTS?

*I*f all these products are so bad for us, how are they allowed to be sold in stores? And if they manage to slip through the cracks and make it to the shelves, aren't they required to carry some sort of warning label so we know exactly what we're signing up for?

Seems practical, right? This is something I hear quite often. It's something I used to believe, and I'm guessing maybe it has crossed your mind as well. We will answer these questions very soon, but first, I want to talk to you about salad dressing. Yes, salad dressing.

If I asked you to name three ingredients in your favourite salad dressing, you could easily answer that because you either make it yourself, or you could check the label on the bottle in your fridge. That magic label lets you know exactly what is in the bottle, and it doesn't leave anything out—because it's not *allowed* to leave anything out. But when it comes to household products, however, that is simply not the case.

Did you know that, unlike food and cosmetics, household cleaning products are not legally required to disclose all their ingredients on the label?[7] The unfortunate truth is that these com-

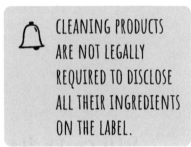
CLEANING PRODUCTS ARE NOT LEGALLY REQUIRED TO DISCLOSE ALL THEIR INGREDIENTS ON THE LABEL.

panies can use any number of ingredients in their products and they don't have to tell us what they are unless they are "chemicals of known concern."

How are they allowed to do this?

Because of a little thing called *trade secrets* law. These are laws that were created to protect companies from unfair competition. Nobody wants to have their products copied and sold as cheap knock-offs, so companies are allowed to claim that their formulas are confidential—a "trade secret."

And that is fair and within their rights. But when companies take advantage and abuse these laws to protect themselves from scrutiny, we as consumers are forced to dig deeper.

Unlisted Ingredients

Let me ask you a question: without knowing exactly what is in your products, can you make informed decisions about what you're bringing into your home? Can you ensure your peace of mind in knowing that you've made the safest choices for your family? Without transparency and a clear list of ingredients, can you ever be sure?

If you're using mainstream cleaning products, you'll be hard-pressed to find anything close to a proper list of ingredients on the label. You might find something like *"contains surfactants"* or *"active ingredient: sodium hypochlorite...2.4%"* but you'll find absolutely nothing about what's in the other 97.6%.

To illustrate my point, imagine if the only thing listed on that bottle of salad dressing was, *"contains lemon juice"* or *"olive oil...52%."* Wouldn't you be concerned about what makes up the rest of the bottle? Would you still pour it all over your salad without knowing for sure? It sounds absurd, but that is exactly what we're doing every time we use any of the dozens of household products we have in our home.

"But Sarah," I hear you saying, "we don't eat our household products, so what's the big deal?"

To which I would respond, dear reader, as we learned in the previous chapter, these products are polluting the very air we breathe. So yes, in a sense, we are still ingesting them after all.

Hidden Ingredients

OK so let's take it one step further because sometimes you do find what looks like a complete list of ingredients on a product label. Even if you don't understand every word, you can see that it's a long list and it seems comprehensive.

Does that mean it's automatically safe to use? Not necessarily. Because apart from unlisted ingredients, there is something else you have to look out for—*hidden* ingredients.

What's the difference between unlisted and hidden? Unlisted ingredients, as we've just seen, are ingredients that were intentionally excluded from the list for one reason or another.

Hidden ingredients, on the other hand, are those that, along with several others, make up a larger umbrella ingredient. So it's one main ingredient listed on the label, when in fact, that one ingredient can be made up of hundreds of sub-ingredients.

A prime example of these umbrella ingredients is the term *fragrance*. There are more than 3,000 fragrance chemicals in use today. But you won't find any of them listed on a label, because their formulations are a "trade secret" (there's that term again). A single fragranced product can contain anywhere from 50 to 300 different fragrance chemicals,[8] but they're all effectively hidden from view because they're listed under that single, ambiguous name—*fragrance*. So even if a label technically lists *fragrance* as an ingredient, it's misleading at best, and deceptive at worst.

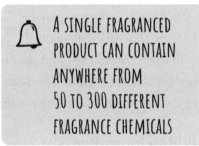

A SINGLE FRAGRANCED PRODUCT CAN CONTAIN ANYWHERE FROM 50 TO 300 DIFFERENT FRAGRANCE CHEMICALS

REMEMBER:

Cleaning products are not legally required to put a complete ingredients list on their label because of "trade secrets" laws. This leads to unlisted, and sometimes hidden ingredients. You wouldn't buy food or cosmetic products under these circumstances, would you? So why allow it for your household products?

Now that we have a little more background on labels and ingredients, let's get back to answering those questions we posed at the beginning of this chapter—about safety and testing.

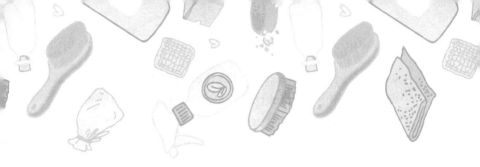

CHAPTER 3:
SAFETY TESTING...
OR A LACK THEREOF

Can I let you in on a little secret? A secret that the cleaning products industry doesn't want you to know about?

Most of the products used around the home in the United States are not legally required to undergo any third-party safety testing or obtain government approval of their formulas before they are bottled and sold on the market. (An exception to this is disinfectants and sanitizers since they are regulated as pesticides, not cleaning products, and therefore they do require prior approval.)[9]

It's bad enough that these companies are allowed to hide what's in their products, but no safety testing or government approval, either? That's just adding insult to injury.

Government Regulation in the US

In the United States, the Environmental Protection Agency (EPA) is in charge of regulating industrial chemicals. This would lead you to believe that these regulators are hard at work banning harmful chemicals from being used in household cleaning products, right? Wrong. Only a small percentage of chemicals are regulated in the United States.

In 1976, the US government passed the Toxic Substances Control Act (TSCA), giving the EPA the authority to regulate the safety of industrial chemicals and to protect human health and the environment. This law was supposed to usher in a new era of proper reporting, testing, and, most importantly, restrictions on chemicals that posed an "unreasonable risk of injury" to our health or the environment.[10]

However, almost from its inception, this law has proven to be ineffective and riddled with flaws. For example, the day the law went into effect, over 60,000 industrial chemicals that were already on the market were grandfathered in and allowed to stay on the market without any further review or testing. Today, there are over 80,000 chemicals used in the US, and most of them have never been tested for safety.[11]

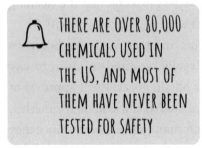

THERE ARE OVER 80,000 CHEMICALS USED IN THE US, AND MOST OF THEM HAVE NEVER BEEN TESTED FOR SAFETY

The Testing Process

So what happens when the EPA wants to test a chemical that they believe might be harmful? Here's where things get tricky. Before the US government will allow them to test a chemical, the EPA has to prove that the chemical poses an "unreasonable risk" to human health. But they can't exactly prove that unless they thoroughly examine and analyze that chemical in the lab.

So the EPA inevitably gets stuck in a catch-22 situation: before they can test a chemical, they have to prove that it poses a risk—but how can they prove that it poses a risk without testing the chemical first?

The process is so long and burdensome that the EPA has ordered testing for fewer than 200 existing chemicals in the last 40 years. For reference, that's .0025% of all chemicals in use today (in the US).[12]

And how many of those were successfully banned? Five. Yes, just five.[13]

New Chemicals Are Under-regulated

What about new chemicals introduced after the 1976 law?

Before a new chemical is brought to market, companies must submit a notice to the EPA outlining "the new chemical's name, physical properties, and use, along with any available data on its toxicity."[14]

But according to a 1998 EPA report, only 7% of the nearly 3,000 "high production volume chemicals" (produced at 1 million pounds or more annually) have a complete set of basic toxicity information. And 43% have no information available at all.[15]

Quite frankly, those numbers shocked me. How can almost half of these high-volume chemicals not have any publicly available safety information?

Again, this is because of the flawed process under which the EPA is forced to operate. Once a company submits its notice for a new chemical, the EPA has just 90 days to make a decision. A decision based on insufficient data and an impossibly tricky testing process. Unfortunately, with limited budgets and resources, too many chemicals are being approved and flooded onto the market without proper testing or regulation.

How the US Differs from Other Countries

It's important to recognize that chemicals are regulated differently in different parts of the world. For example, while the United States takes an "innocent until proven guilty" approach to chemical safety, other countries (like those in the European Union and Canada) operate under what's known as the "precautionary principle."

Ideally, the burden should be on product companies to prove that their products are safe to use. But in the US, the burden falls on individual consumers (or the EPA) to prove that a product or chemical is harmful. That means that if you suspect that your face cream, for example, is the cause of your cystic acne, you would have to take that company to court and prove your claim beyond the shadow of a doubt—an almost impossible feat.

The European Union

This is vastly different from the way things are handled in the EU. The precautionary principle puts the onus on the product companies to prove that the chemicals they use are safe. If there is any suspected harm from a specific chemical, the government will immediately move to regulate or, if necessary, ban that chemical.

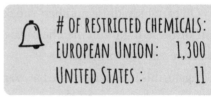

OF RESTRICTED CHEMICALS:
EUROPEAN UNION: 1,300
UNITED STATES :   11

To illustrate what this looks like in action, let's consider a quick example from the cosmetics industry: the EU has restricted or completely banned over 1,300 chemicals in cosmetic products alone.[16] In contrast, the US has only banned 11.[17]

Canada

Canada also employs the precautionary principle for regulating chemicals. The Canadian Environmental Protection Act of 1999 (CEPA) requires all new chemicals, made or imported after 1994, to be assessed against a specific set of criteria before they enter the market.[18]

However, like the US, many of the chemicals in use today (about 23,000) were introduced several decades *before* CEPA went into effect. But that's where the similarities end. Unlike the US, Canada has created a robust process for handling them and, in 2006, became the first country in the world to systematically sort through and categorize the thousands of chemicals in use before their environmental protection laws were created. Because of this, they have been able to identify which chemicals do not require further testing and can focus their efforts on the remaining, high-priority chemicals.[19]

Bridging the Gap

So why the large gap in policies across the globe? It's not exactly clear cut, but some experts believe that this might be related to the issue of government-funded health care.

The US has a privatized healthcare system, meaning its citizens—not the government—are responsible for healthcare costs. The EU and Canada, on the other hand, both have some form of subsidized health care where the government foots the bill. So it's in their interests to regulate the harmful chemicals that can cause chronic health conditions in order to reduce the strain they can put on the healthcare system.

Of course, no system is perfect, and the issue is much more complex than we can cover in this chapter, but it certainly gives us something to think about.

REMEMBER:

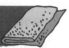

In the United States, most chemicals in production are not properly tested before being released to the market. Nor are they regulated in the way that we would expect. The US treats chemicals as "innocent until proven guilty," while other countries, including Canada and the EU, follow the "precautionary principle." Regardless of their laws, it's our job as consumers to educate ourselves on these chemicals so we can make informed decisions.

We've covered a lot so far—on chemicals, ingredients, and labeling laws. Now that we have a good foundation, we're going to learn how to decipher all those foreign words and symbols we see on the dozens of household products we come across on store shelves.

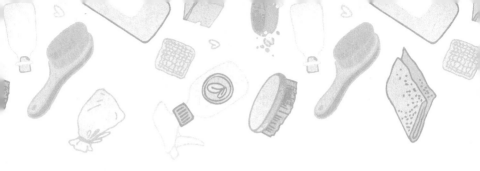

CHAPTER 4:
HOW TO READ LABELS LIKE A BOSS

A ll-natural. Eco-friendly. Sustainable. Organic.
These words are plastered across all sorts of household products at the store. They're supposed to give you assurance and confidence in the safety and quality of these products. But what do they mean for you as a consumer? And can they be trusted at face value? Finding the answers to these questions requires us to read between the lines and get familiar with a tricky thing called *greenwashing*.

What is Greenwashing?

I want you to think back to the last time you stood in a store and compared two or more products, hoping to choose the best one for your family. Without knowing you or the specific products you compared, I can almost guarantee that you most probably picked the one with words like "natural," "non-toxic," or "eco-friendly" on the packaging. Perhaps the label included neutral, earthy tones like greens, browns, and tans. Maybe some leaves or trees, or planet Earth.

But here's the thing: while choosing a product with these features is probably better than not, the truth is that anyone can slap these words on a label without having to prove their claims. Marketing terms like "natural" and "green" are not regulated and have no real meaning when it comes to product safety.[20] They are not verified by a third party, and each company can make up its standards for what these terms mean.

While tricky marketing language may initially grab your attention, remember that the most important part of a product label is what is on the back. So when you're at the store trying to choose the safest products for your family, you always want to flip that bottle around and inspect the details on the back. Because that's where the truly valuable information can be found.

What to Look for on a Label

Ingredients List

First, glance through the ingredients list and see if you can spot any of the Worst Offenders (found in Chapter 5). If you see one of them on the list, you have to decide if that's an ingredient you're willing to allow into your home. For example, if you suffer from asthma or eczema, you'll want to avoid specific ingredients that can aggravate these conditions.

If the product you're looking at does not include a list of ingredients, put it back and choose another one. If the manufacturer hasn't taken the time or effort to provide you with a list of what is in their product, then they don't deserve your business. It's as simple as that.

Exclusions List

Next, look for a list that tells you what is *not* in the product. For example, "contains no phosphates, no bleach, no SLES," etc. While this list is not exhaustive and should not be used on its own, it is still a good starting point and an indicator that a company is paying attention to what they put in their products.

Official Certifications

You'll also want to look for official seals of approval from reputable certifying organizations (see list below). A product with any of these seals has gone through rigorous third-party verification to ensure that at least 70% of its ingredients are certified organic (some of them contain at least 95%).

Organic Organizations

- **USDA Organic**
- **Euro Leaf**
- **Canada Organic**
- **NSF International**
- **Oregon Tilth (OTCO)**
- **Eco Cert**
- **Natrue**

Manufacturers must pay to get their products certified, and if they break the rules, they have to pay a hefty fine. With such strict standards, certified organic products are usually trustworthy. But don't just look for the word "organic" on the label; the product must also bear an official seal to be considered truly organic. This also goes for any food or consumer products. For a complete list of organic certifications from around the world, you can visit: organicandyourhealth.com/organic-product-logo

Besides the organic seals, I do want to bring your attention to two other seals that I trust and highly recommend. The **EWG Verified** and **Made Safe** seals are used for products that follow rigorous verification from these organizations. Products with these seals must be free from any ingredients that are known or suspected to cause human health harm. If you see a product at the store or online with one of these seals, you can be almost 100% sure that they are safe to use for your family.

Where to Find Help

More often than not, when I mention the idea of reading labels and looking at ingredients, I'm met with either blank stares or some form of *"Who has time for all that?"*

Look, I get it—your time is valuable. And the last thing you need while you're out shopping is to spend even more of your already limited time reading big words that most of us don't understand. Seriously, who *does* have time for all of that?

The good news is that nowadays, there are many great resources available to help us get a few steps ahead of the game, so we're not spending hours and hours trying to decipher obscure chemical names. I've spent quite a bit of time digging into these resources over the past few years, and while they do offer some much-needed guidance, sometimes they can be a bit overwhelming.

That's why one of the major aspects of this book—and something I haven't seen much of in other print books—is the lists of Alternative Options included with each household product we'll discuss in Part III when we go through the Room-by-Room Analysis. I've personally curated these after a good deal of cross-referencing various resources to help you find the safest products for your family.

With that being said, I also want you to be empowered with the knowledge you need to read labels confidently on your own, so I'm including a list of the main resources I use to help me choose the best products for my family, in the hope that it helps you do the same for yours.

Consumer Product Organizations

- **Campaign for Safe Cosmetics**
- **Environmental Defence Canada**
- **Safer Chemicals, Healthy Families**
- **EWG Guide to Healthy Cleaning**
- **EWG Skin Deep Database**
- **Made Safe**

> For a list of mobile apps that you can use to scan and analyze specific products while you are at the store, check out the Additional Resources section in the Appendix at the end of this book.

An important thing to note here is that no single organization on this list is the be-all and end-all of consumer product safety. They each have their strengths and weaknesses, so I like to use them all together instead of relying on any single source.

However, if I had to pick just one for you to focus on, it would be the Environmental Working Group (EWG), which has separate databases for cleaning and personal care products.

EWG uses a simple rating system to rate cleaning products on a scale of A-F, and personal care products on a scale of 1-10. In general, you want to stick with products that score an A or B for cleaners, and a 1 or 2 for personal care. These are products that are made with the safest ingredients, free

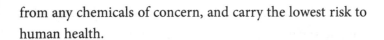

from any chemicals of concern, and carry the lowest risk to human health.

A little caveat...

I do take issue with the way EWG sometimes handles their rating system. It seems that they don't weigh their scores by the concentration of each ingredient (because of trade secrets, as we discussed in Chapter 3). They treat them as if they are all distributed in equal proportions.

Why is this a problem?

Because when you have a chemical that can be harmful when used at full strength but is completely harmless in its diluted form, it's unfair to give it a failing score regardless of how much of it is used in the final product.

An easy example to help illustrate this issue is table salt. We would never take a salt shaker and sprinkle salt directly into our eyes. That would be quite painful and could lead to permanent damage! But many of us have used a saline solution—which is just salt diluted in water to about 1% concentration—to clean or lubricate our eyes. Is it fair, then, to give the saline solution a bad score simply because it contains table salt? Of course not.

Nevertheless, I want you to understand that I am not against the EWG by any means. I believe they have done some amazing work empowering consumers like you and me to make choices that align with our values. I just encourage you to be a little critical and take their ratings...with a grain of salt. (Sorry, I just couldn't resist the pun!)

REMEMBER: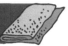

The most important part of a product label is what is on the back. Greenwashing has become ubiquitous and nearly impossible to avoid. But if we know what to look for and where to get help when we need it, we can beat these sneaky companies at their own game.

Are you feeling a little more confident in your knowledge of these issues yet? I hope so because you've made it through the heaviest chapters of this book. The next chapter, while also jam-packed with information, gives us a more practical look at some of the worst chemicals that are used in our household products, and what we can do to reduce our exposure to them.

"

Do the best you can until you
know better. Then when you know
better, do better.

— MAYA ANGELOU

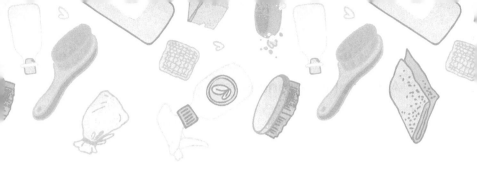

CHAPTER 5:
THE WORST OFFENDERS

You're getting more comfortable with reading product labels, and you're ready to put your new skills to practice. But one look at the back of that cleaning spray bottle, and you're feeling overwhelmed again. That label has over a dozen different ingredients on there! Where do you start? It all seems like too much!

Breathe, my friend. And let's figure it out together. In this chapter, we're going to explore some of the very worst ingredients that you'll want to keep an eye out for, how they can affect your health, and how to spot them in your products so you can avoid them as much as possible.

The recommendations in this chapter are basic guidelines and should be taken as quick and simple action points for areas that you can focus on right away. Choose the ones that are most important to you for your situation—for example, if you have sensitive skin or suffer from asthma—but most of all, do the best you can with what you have.

Artificial Fragrances

As we learned in Chapter 2, the word *fragrance* on an ingredient list is a blanket term for a chemical cocktail that can be made up of any number of the 3,000+ different fragrance chemicals in use today.

Artificial fragrances are some of the most prevalent chemicals found in nearly every type of household product—from cleaners and hair products to children's toys and cosmetics. And although they can smell nice, they have been shown to cause allergic reactions, multiple chemical sensitivities, and respiratory problems, as well as more serious conditions involving the immune and neurological systems.[21]

Remember those volatile organic compounds (VOCs) we talked about earlier? The ones that release harmful particles into the air we breathe? Air fresheners and other products that contain artificial fragrances are loaded with VOCs, so it's best to avoid them as much as you can.

To limit your exposure
- Choose products labelled *fragrance-free*
- Avoid products with *fragrance, natural fragrance,* or *parfum* in the ingredients list
- Choose products that only use pure essential oils or plant extracts for a natural scent

Note: *Unscented* is not the same as *fragrance-free*. Unscented products can still contain fragrance chemicals to mask the scent of the ingredients that are used to make the product. So, remember to always choose fragrance-free!

Phthalates

Another group of chemicals found in artificial fragrances is *phthalates*, which are used to stabilize fragrances and make their scent last longer. They can also be found in pesticides that are used on conventional farms, as well as in some plastic products to make them softer and more pliable.

Phthalates have been linked to health issues like headaches, asthma, and inflammation, as well as more serious concerns like hormone disruption, fertility issues, and some types of cancers (in rats and mice).[22]

To limit your exposure

- Avoid products with artificial fragrances
  (i.e., no *fragrance* or *parfum* in the ingredients list)
- Avoid plastic whenever possible
  (more in Chapters 8 and 9)
- Choose products labeled *PVC-free* or *phthalate-free*
- Avoid recycling code 3, which identifies PVC products
- Eat organic produce, meat, and dairy when possible

Ammonia

Commonly found in nature and also produced by the human body, ammonia is a naturally occurring, highly irritating gas. When dissolved in water, it forms ammonium hydroxide—the main ingredient found in many window cleaners. It is also sold as a standalone cleaning product.

Inhalation of ammonia can cause irritation or burning of the eyes, nose, throat, and respiratory tract.[23]

To limit your exposure

- Avoid products containing *ammonia* or *ammonium hydroxide*, like window cleaners.

Sodium Hypochlorite (Bleach)

Household bleach is used on its own or as a disinfectant in many cleaning products. It should not be mixed with ammonia, vinegar, alcohol, or any acid-based products, as the resulting fumes can be very dangerous or even deadly. Bleach is very good at its job (cleaning and disinfecting) but is not without its risks.

The inhalation of bleach can aggravate asthma and allergies. It is also irritating to the skin, eyes, and respiratory tract. Poorly ventilated rooms can be extra hazardous—especially for children and pets—as the fumes linger in the air and contribute to indoor air pollution.[24]

To limit your exposure
- Avoid products containing *sodium hypochlorite,* including toilet bowl cleaners, scouring powders, and disinfectants.

1,4-dioxane

This one is tricky because you won't find it listed on any ingredients list. That's because it is a by-product of the manufacturing process of some ingredients, which can be found in laundry detergents and other sudsy, foamy products like hand soaps, dish soaps, and shampoos.

The process, called *ethoxylation*, is used to create surfactants (i.e., detergents) by reacting certain chemicals with *ethylene oxide*—which is known to be a human carcinogen, according to the U.S. Department of Health and Human Services.[25] This ethoxylation process can also contaminate these products with *1,4-dioxane,*[26] which the EPA also classifies as a likely human carcinogen.[27]

The only way to remove these contaminants from the affected products is by vacuum stripping them. Some companies have policies in place for handling this process, but you would have to contact each company to check their policy. It should also be noted that this process is completely voluntary, so companies are under no legal obligation to remove these contaminants from their products, which means most of them just skip it.

To limit your exposure

- Avoid ingredients ending with -*eth* and -*oxynol,* like *sodium laureth sulfate, steareth, ceteareth,* and *nonoxynol.*
- Avoid products with *PPG, PEG, polyethylene, polyethylene glycol,* and *polyoxyethylene* in the ingredients list.

Sodium Lauryl Sulfate (SLS) vs. Sodium Laureth Sulfate (SLES)

At first glance, these look very similar—both are detergents, meant to attach themselves to dirt and grease and rinse them away—but the small variation between *lauryl* and *laureth* makes a big difference.

Since SLS can be harsh on the skin, formulators have tried to "soften" it by putting it through the ethoxylation process mentioned above, to create SLES—a much gentler detergent. However, as we just learned, this process can also contaminate the final product with that nasty 1,4-dioxane, so it's best to avoid SLES altogether.

As for SLS, on the other hand, this one is fine to use in cleaning products, as long as they will not come in contact with your skin. In other words, if your dish soap contains SLS, it's best to avoid it, unless you wear dish gloves while washing the dishes; but if your toilet bowl cleaner contains SLS, it's perfectly fine to use since it won't come in contact with your skin.

To limit your exposure

- Avoid any products containing *sodium laureth sulfate* (SLES).
- Avoid *sodium lauryl sulfate* (SLS) in products that come in contact with skin (e.g., hand soap or dish soap).

Quaternary Ammonium Compounds (QACs)

QACs are organic compounds that can be found in a variety of cleaning products, including fabric softeners, disinfectants, and detergents.

In laundry products, they are designed to cling to fabrics—even after they've been rinsed with water—to make them feel softer. That's how fabric softeners work; by coating your fabrics with a thin layer of conditioners that don't rinse off. When used in disinfecting products, QACs are effective against a broad range of viruses and bacteria, but their indiscriminate and widespread use has been found to contribute to antibiotic resistance.[28]

Exposure to QACs can cause skin and respiratory irritation, the most common kind being an allergic reaction called *contact dermatitis*, with symptoms of red, itchy, irritated skin. QACs can also trigger asthma symptoms in people who already have asthma—but what's more alarming is that they can also cause "new onset of asthma in people with **no prior asthma.**"[29] Yikes!

I've said this before, and I'll keep saying it: fabric softeners are terrible for your health and should be one of the very first things you get rid of on this journey.

To limit your exposure

- Avoid fabric softener products.
- Avoid using dryer sheets.
- Avoid disinfectant products like Lysol®.
- Avoid laundry detergents with "built-in" fabric softeners.

Optical Brighteners

Optical brighteners are added to laundry detergents to make fabrics look whiter and brighter. Instead of cleaning or removing stains from fabrics, they absorb ultraviolet light and reflect blue light. These chemicals trick your eyes into thinking your whites are whiter and more vibrant—but it's all just an optical illusion.

Like QACs, optical brighteners are designed to coat your fabrics, so they never get rinsed out. Want to see these chemicals in action? Look at your clothes under a black light; if you notice an unnatural glow, those are the optical brighteners at work!

These brighteners are typically made from benzene, which is highly toxic and does not break down in the environment. And because they get absorbed into fabrics and can rub off onto your skin, the residue left behind may cause allergic reactions when your skin is exposed to sunlight.[30]

To limit your exposure

- Avoid mainstream laundry detergents (refer to the list of safer alternatives in The Laundry Room chapter in Part III)

Triclosan

This antibacterial ingredient is added to soaps, body washes, and dish soaps to help kill germs and prevent bacterial infections. However, the US Food and Drug Administration (FDA) now advises that there isn't enough evidence to show that these products are any better at preventing infection than plain soap and water. Furthermore, there is growing concern over the possibility that long-term exposure to these products could lead to antibiotic resistance (discussed further in Chapter 6).

Because of these new findings, the FDA issued a final rule in 2017 that bans the use of triclosan in over-the-counter products without preliminary review.[31] However, although this ingredient is slowly disappearing from new products, you can still find it in some older products and those sold in dollar stores and outlets.

To limit your exposure
- Avoid products containing *triclosan*, like soaps and washes.
- Avoid soaps and washes labelled as *antibacterial*.

REMEMBER:

You can't completely remove all of these chemicals from your life, but you can control which ones you bring into your home. Start with one or two that you feel would make the most impact on your quality of life and go from there. Looking for a quick win? Start with artificial fragrances since they're the easiest to spot on a label. Many companies are catching on to the fact that we don't want these chemicals in our products, so they now offer fragrance-free versions of their products.

That last offender, triclosan, is a special one because killing germs is an obvious necessity, right? Well, let's talk about germs, shall we? But this discussion deserves its own chapter, so let's continue this chat on the next page.

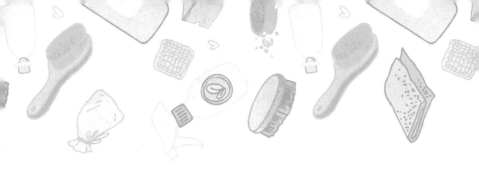

CHAPTER 6:
WHAT ABOUT THE GERMS?

et's face it: germs are horrible, right? They're dangerous, filthy, unhealthy, and some are even deadly! But is that true of all germs? Does every microscopic organism have to be eradicated from the face of the Earth for us to have happy and healthy lives?

The answer, of course, is no. The truth is that we need germs to live. Our bodies are housing billions of them as we speak. The air we breathe, the ground we walk on, the water we drink, and the food we eat—every living thing on this planet would die without the bacteria, viruses, fungi, and other microorganisms present in our natural world.

But one quick stroll down the cleaning aisle of your supermarket would have you believe otherwise. In the last two decades alone, we've seen an unprecedented number of antibacterial products hitting store shelves.

From soaps and cleaners to toothpastes and even facial tissues, manufacturers have jumped at the opportunity to feed and play on our fears about disease and hygiene. We're convinced that we need the latest and greatest products to kill "99.9%" of all bacteria.

But at what cost?

Of course, antibacterial products have their place in society; they were originally used exclusively in hospitals and other healthcare settings where the risk of infection is disproportionately high. Also, households with elderly people or those with compromised immune systems would surely benefit from a highly sanitized environment.

But the vast majority of households do not need to be sterile, and there's a growing body of evidence showing that the overuse of these products is causing more harm than good. In our efforts to eradicate all germs from our homes—an impossible feat, of course—our incessant use of antibacterial products has led to a significant rise in the prevalence of antibiotic-resistant bacteria. These are bacteria that have mutated over time to create new, more dangerous strains that are now resistant to antibiotics.[32]

Remember, antibacterial products don't just kill the scary germs; they kill *all* germs— even the good ones that our bodies need to stay healthy. These products are changing the delicate

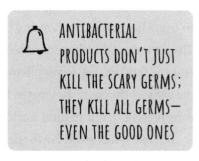

ANTIBACTERIAL PRODUCTS DON'T JUST KILL THE SCARY GERMS; THEY KILL ALL GERMS— EVEN THE GOOD ONES

balance of healthy and unhealthy bacteria in our bodies, which can lead to an immune system imbalance.

How This Affects Our Immune System

Our immune system needs to be exposed to all kinds of germs throughout our life so it can learn to fight off infections. But if our homes and immediate environments are constantly over-sanitized, then the immune system doesn't get the exposure it needs to develop properly. Then, when we eventually do get exposed to harmful germs, our body isn't ready to fight back because it wasn't properly trained to do so. It's like showing up for a championship boxing match without ever having set foot in a gym. The odds are stacked against us.

Autoimmune & Allergic Diseases

So what do you think happens to the immune system when it's not getting enough germ-fighting action? How does it cope with the boredom that comes with not being able to do its job? After all, if the immune system was specifically designed to attack harmful bacteria, what does it do when there's nothing around to attack?

Well, without an adequate supply of those foreign invaders, sometimes the immune system gets confused and does the unthinkable: it can turn on itself and start attacking the body's healthy cells, tissues, and organs. This self-sabotaging behaviour can lead to autoimmune diseases like type 1 diabetes, Hashimoto's disease, multiple sclerosis (MS), and rheumatoid arthritis.[33]

Another common immune disorder—asthma—has also been linked to the use of household cleaning products. One international study concluded that these products—specifically those in spray form—could be an important risk factor for adult asthma.[34] Although these findings are preliminary and need to be confirmed with further studies, they may have serious implications for public health.

It's no secret that autoimmune diseases and asthma—especially among young children—have increased dramatically in recent years. What's interesting is that this increase is directly correlated with a decrease of certain bacteria in the home.[35] Again, our homes are becoming "too clean" for our immune systems to develop properly, especially in the early years of life.

But let's be clear about something here since correlation does not imply causation. Am I saying that the use of antibacterial products leads to autoimmune and allergic diseases? No, of course not. What I am saying is that if someone is already genetically predisposed to one of these diseases, long-term exposure to antibacterial products could be one of many factors in triggering the onset of an autoimmune or allergic disease.

Just Use Soap and Water

Seriously, that's all we need. Plain soap and water. Not antibacterial soap; just regular soap. All the major health organizations—including the World Health Organization, the Centres for Disease Control and Prevention, and Health Canada—agree that the first line of defence against bacteria and viruses should be good hand-washing practices and that antibacterial products like hand sanitizers should only be used when soap and water are not readily available.

This advice has been at the forefront of the COVID-19 global pandemic as one of the most effective ways to stop the spread of the virus.[36]

What about Essential Oils?

Essential oils seem to be everywhere nowadays and for good reason. Not only are they great for aromatherapy and cleaning and freshening the air, many oils have also been shown to have significant antibacterial and antifungal activity.[37] But not only that; in-vitro studies have also shown essential oils to be a practical option for preventing infections from antibiotic-resistant bacteria.[38] In other words, when bacteria mutate and become resistant to antibiotics, essential oils can be a promising alternative to treat those bacterial infections.

For a list of common essential oils that you can use in your cleaning routine, as well as some trusted brands that I recommend, please refer to the "Essential Oils for Cleaning" section in the Appendix.

Finding the Balance

Look, I'm not advocating that we allow germs to overtake our living spaces and roam free, uncontrolled and unchecked, just like I'm not suggesting that we douse our homes in bleach to exterminate every last germ.

I'm only challenging you to reconsider the narrative we've all been playing in our minds. The one that says our homes are not clean if they're not completely disinfected. (They are.) The one that insists that proper handwashing with soap and water is not enough these days. (It is.) And the one that has us convinced that we need stronger and stronger chemicals to truly feel safe in our own homes. (We don't.)

In the previous chapter, we touched on some of the most harmful chemicals found in common cleaning products, including those that promise to kill 99.9% of bacteria. And if the side effects and health issues associated with them haven't urged you to think twice about using them in your home, then I invite you to at least give some thought to the long-term effects these products have on our immune systems and those of our children and grandchildren.

REMEMBER:

Am I saying you should never use antibacterial products? No, absolutely not. They have their place and time; we just need to be more mindful and prudent about when, where, and how we use them if we want to live in a healthy balance with our environment.

You've made it to the end of Part I of this book, how exciting! We've gotten through quite a bit of information so far. All of which is necessary to get you prepped and ready for the next step—getting started on your journey! It's time for some interactive, hands-on, action-based work, you guys. On to Part II!

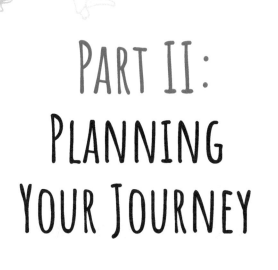

Part II:
Planning
Your Journey

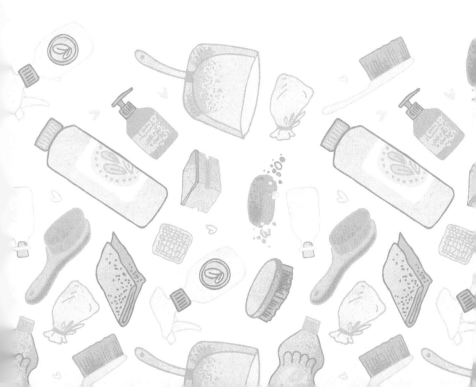

"

He who has a why can endure
any how.

— FREDERICK NIETZCHE

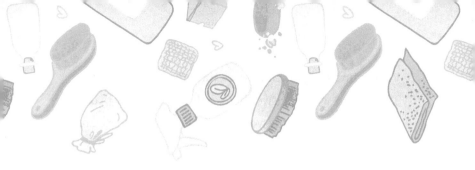

CHAPTER 7:

DISCOVERING YOUR "WHY"

N ow that you have a good, solid foundation for your home, you're ready to build the frame that will keep it standing in the face of whatever obstacles may arise on your journey. Obstacles like self-doubt, failure, and unforeseen circumstances. But without a clear sense of purpose—without knowing your "Why"—that frame will buckle under the slightest bit of pressure.

In this chapter, you're going to discover your Why Statement. This intentional statement will help you focus your efforts on what matters most and push you forward whenever you feel like giving up. It's what will carry you through and help you stay on this journey for the long haul, no matter what comes your way.

Now I want you to take a moment and read the three simple statements below. Then go ahead and rank them in order of importance, with "1" being the most important to you, and "3" being the least important:

____ I want to protect my family's health and well-being.

____ I want to live a more eco-friendly and sustainable lifestyle.

____ I want to save money and be more self-sufficient.

Which one did you choose as the most important?

There is no wrong answer here, only the one that makes the most sense for you and your family. Of course, these are just suggestions to get you thinking about your purpose on this journey, so if you come up with something different, that's great! As long as it speaks to you and you can fully own it.

> **Think about it**: Why is it that you want to be on this journey to a non-toxic home? What aspirations do you have for your family? Visualize what this journey looks like for you, and what lies at the end of the road. What are you travelling towards? What is your goal? What exactly are you trying to achieve?

Once you've discovered your Why Statement, go ahead and write it down somewhere, and make it your mantra for this journey. That way you can come back to it when you hit dead-ends or bumps in the road, like self-doubt and perceived failure.

I say "perceived" because I don't believe in failure—only mistakes. You see, the road to success is filled with mistakes. But mistakes are not permanent; they're simply opportunities for growth and change. They give you a chance to reassess and improve. To rework your strategy and progress even further toward your goal.

But how, exactly, do you do that? There is a great quote from author and poet, Vironika Tugaleva, in her book, *The Art of Talking To Yourself*:

> *"One thing is for sure—you will make mistakes. Learn to learn from them. Learn to forgive yourself. Learn to laugh when everything falls apart because, sometimes, it will."*

You see, it's not about whether or not you fall (because you will); it's about how you pick yourself up and keep moving. Keep pushing. Keep growing. Because mistakes and slip-ups? They're just part of the process. But they're not the end of the process. And they definitely do not define your journey.

That's why I'm encouraging you to write down your Why Statement and put it somewhere visible. Because those difficult days—those mistake-filled days—are going to happen. They're inevitable, and that's OK. But if you can go back to your purpose—your *Why*—and use that as your guide, then you'll have exactly what you need to proactively turn those mistakes into moments of growth.

Here Is My Why

I grew up in a standard North American household; we didn't pay much attention to product labels or the ingredients in our food, and we sure as heck didn't question what we were using in our homes and on our bodies. Like many others, I lived in this naive state throughout much of my young adult life.

If the government allows these products to be on the shelves and sold to the public, surely they must be safe, I thought. And that's mostly true; except, as we learned in Part I of this book, cleaning products, in particular, are held to different labelling and safety standards.

Then one day, in my mid-twenties, I noticed that my hands started breaking out in itchy, dry, cracked patches that were extremely painful and severely affected my quality of life. After consulting with a dermatologist, I learned that this was a combination of eczema and dermatitis.

What was going on? Why was this happening? And how do I make this stop?

I had so many questions, but my doctor couldn't tell me why I had developed this painful skin condition; she only suggested that I start using prescription medications, including steroid creams, to help manage the flare-ups.

I knew I didn't want to use such strong medicines forever—especially if I didn't even know the cause of these symptoms—so I set out to answer these questions for myself. And this is what jump-started my personal journey of non-toxic living. I started by switching to more natural hand soap and hand lotion, which did reduce the flare-ups but didn't completely get them under control.

Two years later, pregnant with my first child, Yusuf, I found myself in a similar situation—questioning everything I knew about the products I used in my home. I felt overwhelmed. Worried. Helpless at the thought of exposing my precious baby to harmful chemicals. I knew I had to do things differently, but I had no idea where to start.

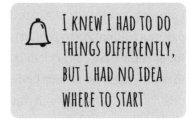

I KNEW I HAD TO DO THINGS DIFFERENTLY, BUT I HAD NO IDEA WHERE TO START

I spent the following years learning, researching, and experimenting with different products and recipes to figure out what works and what doesn't. I came up with roadmaps and formulas to help make the journey easier and more efficient. And slowly but surely, I've examined and replaced nearly all of the products I use in my home, which has, in turn, helped me manage my eczema and get it under control.

Since then, I've taught this method to dozens of families who now have confidence and peace of mind on their path to a safer, healthier home. They're in control of their immediate environment; not because they have a 100% non-toxic home (spoiler alert: that doesn't actually exist), but because they know how to make smarter choices, how to prioritize what's important to them, and what is non-negotiable for them.

I want to help you do the same. So here's what I need you to do right now. Go back and read your Why Statement one more time. Let it sink in. Let it marinate. Give it a cozy spot in your brain because you're going to come back to it again and again.

REMEMBER:

To make progress on your journey, you need a clear sense of purpose. Your Why Statement is meant to give you clarity and help you focus on what's important, so you can always get back up after you fall.

Now that you've zeroed in on your goals and purpose, I want to help you with one more thing before we get into the actual planning of your journey—and that's your mindset.

"

What you're supposed to do when
you don't like a thing is change it.
If you can't change it, change the
way you think about it.

— Maya Angelou

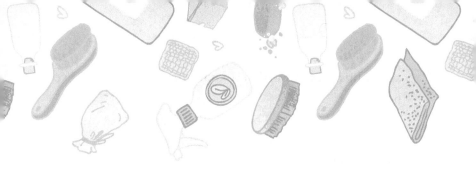

CHAPTER 8:
SHIFTING YOUR MINDSET

This might be the most important chapter you'll read in this book. It's not loaded with facts and figures or action items, but it focuses on what I truly believe can either make or break this journey for you.

I'm going to guess that you have most likely dabbled in the world of natural living before ever picking up this book. Maybe you even started making some small changes here and there. And you started strong. You put in the time, you did the research, and you read all the blogs. You saved some DIY recipes, and maybe you've gone as far as buying all the products, tools, and ingredients because you know this is what you want for your family.

But then, somewhere along the way, you got stuck. And for one reason or another, you just can't seem to make any progress. You're busy with life's demands. You don't have the time or energy to dedicate to this. You don't know where to start, or even how to start. And some days you're not sure if any of this is even worth it. I know the feeling because I've been there.

But here's the thing: before you can get unstuck and get going on this journey, there's something you need to remember. A simple, yet critical, truth:

**You deserve a safe, healthy, natural home
for your family.**

That's right, you *deserve* it. Your family deserves it, your health deserves it, and our planet deserves it. Too often, we sabotage our lofty dreams because deep down, underneath the planning, the research, and the late nights of poring over blog posts and articles, we don't think we deserve what we're dreaming of. There's a little voice in our head telling us we're not worth the effort, or the time, or the energy that it takes to fulfill those dreams.

But I'm calling BS.

Because that little voice? It's lying to you. Just like it has lied to me and countless others just like us. You don't have to listen to that voice. You don't have to let it define you. You have the power—and, dare I say, permission—to tell that little voice to go fly a kite. We don't have time for it.

I'd love to tell you that this journey will be all rainbows and butterflies, and everything will work out effortlessly. But I'd be lying through my teeth.

The fact of the matter is that this new path will have its challenges. Some parts will be hard. Others will be smooth sailing. So if you go into this journey without shifting your mindset, you're bound to be disappointed and disheartened at some point. But if you can keep a few inconvenient truths in mind, you'll be much better prepared to handle those challenges when they arise.

Inconvenient Truths About Non-Toxic Products

1. **They're not as strong as conventional products.** Safer chemicals, by their nature, are gentler, but I'd argue that most of these products don't need to be as potent as we've been used to. Stronger is not always better.

2. **They can be more expensive.** This is a standard example of getting what you pay for. When you use better quality ingredients, they're going to cost more to produce, and the price of the final product will reflect that. But depending on your Why Statement, there's a solution to that.

3. **They require more scrubbing or "elbow grease."** Because they're made with gentle ingredients, sometimes they can take a little longer to work. But this is only true for a few specialty products. Most of the time, this isn't the case.

4. **Their fragrances don't last as long.** Without the harmful additives that make artificial fragrances so strong and long-lasting, natural products just can't compete in this area. But with time, you will learn to accept this reality and prefer the more subtle, delicate scents of natural products. Again, stronger is not always better.

5. **They're not always available at your local store.** Although natural products are becoming more commonplace, they can still be hard to find in some areas. Thankfully, there are lots of online options to fill this gap. (There's a list of stores and websites for you in the Appendix.)

As we can see, there are some things to consider on this journey. But I think you can agree that they're not necessarily deal-breakers, and simply being aware of them beforehand makes them easier to manage down the line.

REMEMBER:

You deserve a safe, healthy, natural home for your family, and it's your job to remind yourself of this whenever you forget. This journey comes with challenges, but if you make a small shift to your mindset and manage your expectations, you'll be much better equipped to handle those challenges with stride.

Alright, now let's switch gears a bit because this next chapter is going to be jam-packed with information. I need you to be ready because I'm laying out the whole roadmap and walking you through the exact formula that I've used for myself and my students over the years. Let's do this.

LEVEL UP YOUR JOURNEY!

We put together some amazing **Bonus Content** just for you! Visit **naturesnurtureblog.com/book** to access the complete library of bonus content that accompanies this book!

Here's what you'll get:

- Printables
- Direct Web Links
- Cheat Sheets
- Recipe Labels
- Checklists
- Reference Cards
- And more!

naturesnurtureblog.com/book

"

Success is a journey,
not a destination.

— BEN SWEETLAND

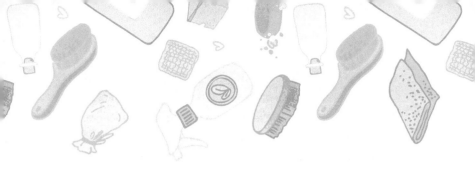

CHAPTER 9:
The Roadmap for Success

E very journey needs a map. Something to keep you grounded, to consult with when you're feeling lost. Something to help you navigate the twists and turns, the unexpected road-blocks, and the inevitable pit stops along the way.

In this chapter, you're going to familiarize yourself with the Roadmap for Success. I developed this over many years while working with families from all over the world. It's worked for large families, newlywed couples, single parents, young bachelors, retired seniors—you name the demographic, and I've probably worked with them.

The philosophy behind this roadmap will become the guiding light of your journey. Over the next few pages, I'll break down each phase of the roadmap and show you exactly how it works and how it all fits together.

ROADMAP FOR SUCCESS	
Phase 1: **Room-by-Room** **Analysis**	We're going to walk through your house together, room by room. I'll point out specific areas to focus on, and we'll tackle them together, one product at a time.
Phase 2: **The Small Steps** **Formula™**	This is the exact formula I've used on my own journey and the one I teach my students. It's the answer to your overwhelm, uncertainty, and whatever is holding you back. Trust me—it works.
Phase 3: **Alternative** **Options**	For each product you want to replace, I'll give you a few different options to choose from—both homemade and store-bought—to help you make the best choice for your family.

Phase 1: The Room-by-Room Analysis

Years ago, when I did one-on-one coaching with families, I was on the phone with a young woman (we'll call her "Angie") who said something that has stuck with me ever since:

"I wish you could jump through the phone and just walk me through this process in person."

And you know what? I wished the same because Angie was struggling at the time. She was a young mom with two small children, and she worked part-time while her mother watched the kids. She wanted so badly to detox her home, especially since she had toddlers who were getting into everything.

But she felt stressed out and defeated. Money was tight, time was tight, and she was living in survival mode most of the time. Thankfully, we continued working together over the phone and got Angie to a comfortable place on her journey. But her comment planted a seed in my brain.

What if I *could* jump through the phone, into Angie's home, and walk through every room of the house with her? Showing her *exactly* what to focus on, how to fix it, and what to use instead?

And that's how the Room-by-Room Analysis was born!

When we get to that section of the book, we're going to go on a virtual walk-through of your entire home. Just imagine that you've invited me over for coffee, and we're casually strolling through your house together—room by room.

Here's how it works

For each room in your home, I'll point out the most important products/areas to focus on, and how you can replace them with a safer alternative—whether that's a homemade version with a recipe or a natural product you can buy at the store instead.

For example, we'll start in the kitchen and do a quick scan to look at everything from your cleaning products to your food storage and explore your options for replacing them. Then we'll move on and repeat the process in the bathroom, the laundry room, and finally, the common living areas.

Once we've scanned your whole house, you'll have a much better idea of what you're working with and what direction you'll take on your journey. I encourage you to skim through all the rooms with me *before* diving in and getting started. It's important to view the lay of the land first so you're clear on which rooms you want to focus on and how you'll prioritize everything. Don't worry, there's also an Action Plan and a Quick Start Guide in the Appendix to help you with this part.

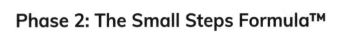

Phase 2: The Small Steps Formula™

Can I let you in on a little secret? Not everyone who starts their non-toxic journey will succeed. Many of them will get overwhelmed, frustrated, and give up entirely.

But you know what? A lot of these defeats are tied to one thing: doing too much, too soon, and all at once. It's normal human behaviour—when we first start learning about dangerous chemicals, unsafe products, and how everything is affecting our health, the natural reaction is to take a giant garbage bag and stuff it with every household product we can find because *"that stuff is going to kill us! Get rid of it… all of it!"*

And that's the moment. The moment that failure rears its ugly head, taunting and mocking you. Because here's another thing about us humans: when we take on too much too fast, we might start strong and determined but we eventually fizzle out, crashing and burning. If that happens enough times, it becomes harder and harder to get back up again.

So if you think you need to throw out all your cleaning products or empty every cupboard in your house before you start this journey, I implore you to stop right there. I strongly advise *against* doing that, because apart from a few exceptions, it can truly be a recipe for disaster.

That's where The Small Steps Formula™ comes in. After years of trial and error on this path, I took everything I learned and came up with a very simple formula to help you start your journey on the right foot. Without the overwhelm. Without stress. And without losing your sanity in the process.

THE SMALL STEPS FORMULA™	
Step 1	Pick **ONE** room in your home that you want to focus on. Is it your kitchen? Your laundry room? Maybe your bathroom?
Step 2	Pick **ONE** product in that room that you want to find a safer alternative for. Is it your dish soap? Your laundry detergent? Your toilet cleaner?
Step 3	Decide if you'll **MAKE** it or **BUY** it. Maybe you're into DIY or on a tight budget. Maybe you're strapped for time, or would rather just buy it from the store. Do what works best for your family.
Step 4	Focus on that **ONE** product (and nothing else!) for as long as it takes for you to find a safer alternative that you're truly happy with (or close enough).
Step 5	Then, and only then, **MOVE ON** to the next product/room that you want to work on. That could be another product in the same room, or a different room entirely.

The Small Steps Formula™ is my solution to the overwhelm. Instead of throwing out all your products and starting from scratch, this method gives you the freedom to gradually convert your home, **one product at a time**. And because you set your own pace, you can work as quickly as you want. Or you can choose to slow it down and take your time with it. It's up to you.

Here's how it works

Because we're naturally inclined to take large tasks and break them down into smaller, more manageable pieces, this formula is broken down into five basic steps—each of which helps you work through the different rooms and products in your home. Let's take a look at how it works.

You're reading this book because you want to create a non-toxic home, so that would be your large task: creating a non-toxic home.

To break this down into smaller tasks, you'll split your home into individual rooms and pick ONE room to focus on (this is step 1). Then you'll look at that room in terms of individual products, and pick ONE product (step 2). So far, so good? Alright, this is where the fun (but also the work) begins. Because now you get to choose which path you'll take: MAKE it or BUY it (step 3).

Do you want to make a homemade version of that product? If you're on a budget or you love to DIY, then that would make the most sense here. But what if you're short on time, or can't be bothered with recipes and ingredients and step-by-steps? Then you'll probably want to look for a safer version that you can buy at the store. Or maybe you start by trying a few recipes, but none of them work for you, so now you want to check out what's available in stores. Everyone's situation and needs are different, so choose what works best for you, remember to be flexible, and give yourself some grace.

Now step 4 is probably the hardest step of this whole formula. Not because it's necessarily difficult to do, but because sometimes we grow impatient, or we lose interest, or quite frankly, we become bored. This step asks you to focus on the ONE product you chose—and nothing else!—for as long as it takes you to find a safer alternative that you're truly happy with.

That means if you're working on switching out your glass cleaner, for example, but you're not impressed with the homemade version you tried, you don't just give up and move on to find a floor cleaner instead. You have to stick it out and push through until you can settle on a glass cleaner that you'll actually use. Because if you don't, you might wake up one day and find a whole bunch of mediocre products that you kind of hate, instead of just a handful of awesome products that you love.

Which would you choose?

> 🔔 YOU MIGHT WAKE UP ONE DAY AND FIND A WHOLE BUNCH OF MEDIOCRE PRODUCTS THAT YOU KIND OF HATE, INSTEAD OF JUST A HANDFUL OF AWESOME PRODUCTS THAT YOU LOVE

A little caveat here: I've been known to have several product experiments going on at the same time, so I guess I don't follow my own advice that well. Eventually, once you've gotten your footing, you can afford to bend the rules a little as well. But when you're first starting out, I do recommend that you stick with the "one product at a time" approach. It's easier, safer, and has a much better success rate.

Phase 3: Alternative Options

I have a younger cousin who's like a sister to me. We grew up together, lived together, and even shared a room during our awkward teen years. She's a wonderful dentist now and is married with three small children, so she's a busy lady. This part of the roadmap, Alternative Options, was entirely inspired by her.

Why?

Because when she got married and had a home of her own to care for, she would call me up at random times of the day, asking for advice on non-toxic products, and the conversation would always end with her asking, flat out:

"Sarah, can you just tell me exactly what to buy?"

That's all she wanted. Guidance on what to buy. She didn't want an explanation of why certain products weren't safe, or a detailed review of the ingredients in other products, or even a simple recipe that would take less than two minutes to whip up.

Nope. She doesn't have time to bother with all of that. All she needed was specific suggestions for safe, non-toxic products that would meet her needs. Nothing more, nothing less. This is why the Alternative Options are now a foundational pillar in the Roadmap for Success—because I know my cousin is not the only one who needs them.

Look, I get it. I know how important it is to balance safety with convenience. And sometimes it's just easier to buy something ready-made from the store instead of mixing it up in your kitchen. I do it all the time, and there's nothing wrong with that.

In fact, we're truly blessed nowadays to have so many safe options available to us. When I started this work back in 2010, those options were few and far between! So this part of the job is always exciting for me because I love learning about new brands that make great products and then sharing them with you to make your life a little easier.

Here's how it works

When we do the Room-by-Room Analysis in Part III of this book, you'll find a list of Alternative Options for each product that we focus on. They are included right after each DIY recipe that I'll share with you, so you won't need to go flipping through different sections of the book. It's all right there in one place.

I've personally handpicked each product—after researching and vetting its ingredients list—to make sure I'm only recommending products that I would use in my own home.

There are a handful of products (oven cleaner, for example) that don't have a list of safer alternatives. That's because I haven't been able to find one yet. In that case, your only option currently is to use the DIY recipe that I've included. But this only applies to a few products. The rest of them have both a recipe (sometimes more than one!) as well as a list of safer store-bought options.

And if you're wondering where exactly you can buy these products, I've also included a list of stores and websites that you can find in the Appendix at the end of this book.

REMEMBER:

The Roadmap for Success has three phases, the most important of which is The Small Steps Formula. Follow it in the order it's laid out, and you'll be set for success on your journey to a non-toxic home.

We're almost ready to jump into Part III and kick off the Room-by-Room Analysis, but there's one last thing we need to cover before we do that. It's incredibly important, especially if you have family members or housemates who aren't necessarily keen on this whole "non-toxic living" idea you keep chiming on about. If that sounds even a tiny bit like your current situation, this next chapter is just for you!

"

Yesterday I was clever,
so I wanted to change the world.
Today I am wise,
so I am changing myself.

— RUMI

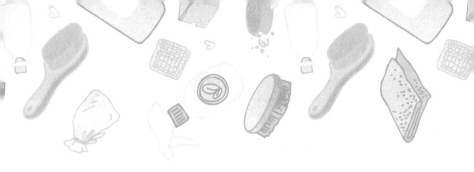

CHAPTER 10:

GETTING YOUR FAMILY ON BOARD

When I started my non-toxic journey, I was the oddball in my family. Nobody understood why I spent so much time reading labels and comparing cleaning products, of all things. I tried teaching them and explaining the reasons behind my new obsession, but my words always fell on deaf ears.

Nobody wanted to hear it. Ignorance is bliss, as they say.

But I'm passionate about this work, so I became even more determined to convert them. It was a long, frustrating process that sometimes ended in toxic debates, loud confrontations, and awkward encounters. Eventually, in order to save our relationships, we became really good at ignoring the issue and carrying on with our own lives. Live and let live.

Thankfully, with lots of time and effort, my family ultimately came around and slowly embraced this lifestyle—be it fully or to a certain extent. Or at the very least, some of them just accept me now as the slightly eccentric hippy who always seems to be whipping up a strange concoction in her kitchen. I'll take it. You can't win them all. But it wasn't easy, and it didn't happen overnight.

Nowadays, when I poll my readers asking them what their biggest struggle is with creating a non-toxic home, I'm always surprised at the number of responses that complain about this same thing: getting their family on board.

I've read email after email, mostly from women, lamenting their struggles with convincing their family members to use safer products.

"Nobody in my house is cooperating," writes one woman.

"My family keeps bringing the toxins in," cries another.

"Others just don't see things the way I do," replies yet another.

And my personal favourite, "They think natural products are dangerous and don't really kill germs."

But nothing compares to the responses I receive from women writing about one specific member of their family— their husband. I would say more than half of the answers I receive for my poll fall into this category:

"My husband just loves bleach!"

"My man is just not into it and continues to use the toxic stuff."

"My husband keeps buying the old stuff when I'm not around."

"I can't convince him that natural products clean better and are better for our health."

To be honest, reading these emails over and over again is emotionally exhausting. I feel for these women. I wish I could reach through my screen, give them a big hug, and tell them that everything will be OK. That they're doing an amazing job, and I'm so proud of them. But comforting words can only go so far. What these women need is practical, actionable advice they can implement right away. So this chapter is dedicated to these awesome women.

Some Tips for Converting Reluctant Family Members

1. Teach what you know

When introducing the idea of non-toxic living to your family, make it very clear what "non-toxic" means to you and how you define it. It helps when they understand that it's not an all-or-nothing deal. So be practical, meet them where they are, and let them see that you're not out to flip their whole world upside down (at least not just yet!).

Share your knowledge with them in a way that matches their learning styles. Your partner may enjoy reading research papers, so send him a short article that you think would resonate and gets your point across. Your mother, on the other hand, might get more out of a discussion with you. Maybe even turn it into a friendly debate. Or maybe your teenager loves to watch movies, so you can pick a documentary, grab some popcorn, and make a movie date out of it!

Check the Appendix at the end of this book for a list of recommended books, websites, and documentary films to get you started.

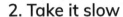

2. Take it slow

It's easy to get excited about everything you learn and want to shout it from the rooftops for everyone to hear. Do NOT do this with your reluctant family members; it just makes them run in the opposite direction (ask me how I know!). Instead, try to ration that knowledge and give them tiny but impactful nuggets that they can think about and digest over a few days.

Likewise, when making changes in your home, remember The Small Steps Formula™ and take it one step, one product, at a time. If you do too much too fast, they'll quit before they even start. But if they only have to commit to changing one thing, your family members are much more likely to cooperate.

3. Make it short-term

Try beginning this journey with your family as a trial run. No commitments. No pressure. If they know there's an endpoint and they can go back to their old ways when it's over, they'll be more likely to give it a shot. You can even make it fun and turn it into a four-week challenge! If you give them some leeway, you might be surprised at the result.

4. Have a plan

Before bringing others on board, always start with a plan. There is a simple Action Plan in the Appendix of this book that you can use for yourself, and then adapt to use with your family. Be clear and honest about what you expect and what is practical for your family. What works for some will not work for others. Include them in the planning and ask for their input so they feel a sense of ownership on this journey.

5. Remember your WHY

Most importantly, relax and enjoy the journey. It has its ups and downs, but if you go back to that Why Statement, you can use it to centre yourself and remember why you started in the first place.

REMEMBER:

At the end of the day, you cannot control other people's actions. You can only control how you respond to them. Lead by example, and the rest may follow. And if they don't, then you have to come to terms with and accept that reality. Be prepared to compromise and find a good balance. For example, my mom uses two different laundry detergents at her house—one for her clothes, and another for her husband's—because he still believes that his clothes aren't truly clean unless they have that strong laundry smell. Balance.

Guess what? We're officially at the end of Part II of the book! And you what that means? Now we get to go furnish your home with safer products. I hope you're excited because I'm pumped and ready to roll. Let's go, my friend.

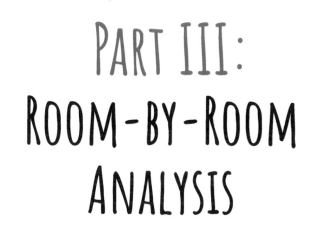

PART III:
ROOM-BY-ROOM
ANALYSIS

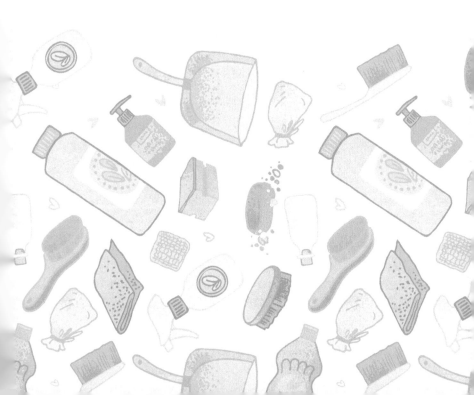

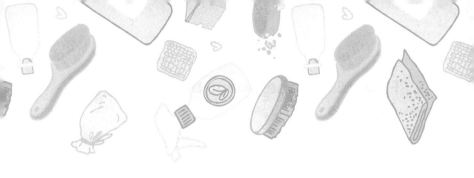

We have finally reached the most fun and exciting part of our journey together! The foundation has been laid, the walls and the roof are up, and now it's time to choose how you're going to furnish your home with safer products for your family.

One quick note before you dig into this section: please remember that the product spotlights in the following chapters are just suggestions and guidelines for what you might consider replacing on your journey. They are in no way meant to make you feel obligated to tackle every single product on the list. Think of them as a menu of options, instead of a rigid list of tasks that must be checked off at any cost.

Likewise, you are not expected to choose a homemade version for every product that you replace—unless that's what you want. We are blessed to have an abundance of alternative options that we can purchase from the store, so use them if and when you need to. The do-it-yourself world is not for everyone, and that's fine. I make many of the products I use in my home, but there is a good handful that I choose to buy instead. Find your balance and work with that.

How to Use the Room-by-Room Analysis

This part of the book is split into four chapters, each of which corresponds to a different room/area of your home:

- **The Kitchen**
- **The Bathroom**
- **The Laundry Room**
- **The Living Areas**

Each chapter begins with an introduction, a list of all the products we will focus on, and a spotlight page for every product in that list. Each spotlight page includes:

- a simple recipe (sometimes more than one!) for making a safer homemade version
- and on the following page is a list of Alternative Options that you can readily buy from a local store or online.

Cleaning Recipes

The recipes in this book are simple, and most of them require just a handful of ingredients that you probably already have at home. The ingredients are listed in both metric and imperial measurements for your convenience. Many recipes also include, where applicable:

- helpful tips for best results
- usage instructions
- safety warnings

Water Warning

You'll also notice in recipes that call for water, I recommend that you use distilled water because it has been purified of any contaminants and, therefore, will greatly extend the shelf life of your products. You can find distilled water sold in gallon jugs at any major grocery store.

If you choose not to use distilled water, you can use plain tap water that has been boiled and cooled. This part is very important; I've had terrible experiences with cleaning products going bad because I just used water straight out of the tap. Water naturally has minerals and bacteria in it, and when you add other ingredients to it, bottle it up, and let it sit in a cupboard for weeks, you could end up with an unwanted science experiment.

Trust me on this one. Distilled water is best. Boiled water is an acceptable alternative, and straight tap water is fine for products that will be used the same day or stored for no more than a couple of weeks.

Alternative Options

I've tried, to the best of my ability, to include alternative options from different regions of the world, including North and South America, Europe, Africa, Asia, and Oceania. So whether you're in Canada like me, the UK, Malaysia, or South Africa, you should be able to find options that are available in your region, either locally or online.

If you're searching for low-waste options, look for (LW) noted after the brand name. And in an effort to support Black-owned businesses, I've highlighted those options as well.

Ingredient Audits

In completing the ingredient audits—yes, I reviewed the ingredients for every single one of the products I recommend in this section, plus the dozens more that didn't make the cut—I followed a simple set of guidelines for choosing the products to include:

1. Full ingredients disclosure on company website is a must.
2. No ambiguous or generic terms in the ingredients list.
3. No synthetic/artificial fragrances allowed. Essential oils are OK.
4. Absolutely no ingredients from the Worst Offenders list allowed.

Where to Find Them

Suggestions for stores and websites that you can purchase these products from are included in the Appendix. I've also included each brand's website address here in the Room-by-Room Analysis so you can visit them online and either order from them directly or find out where you can purchase their products locally.

Sometimes a safer Alternative Option is not available (e.g., for oven cleaner); in that case, I'll indicate this by adding a small note at the bottom of the recipe page.

Side Note

The recommendations in this section are current at the time of publication, but brands and manufacturers can change their products, formulas, or websites at any time. For the most up-to-date listing of Alternative Options—that is revised and updated regularly—please see the Shopping Guide on my website at this link: naturesnurtureblog.com/shop

REMEMBER:

As you go through each room, make some quick mental notes on a few specific products that you would like to concentrate on as you begin your journey. Don't worry about writing them down just yet; we'll get to that later when you fill out your Action Plan. For now, just keep them in mind as you move through each room so you have an idea of what you're working with.

Alright, now grab your favourite drink (I've got my coffee in hand), and let's visit your kitchen!

"

The kitchen really is the castle itself. This is where we spend our happiest moments and where we find the joy of being a family.

— MARIO BATALI

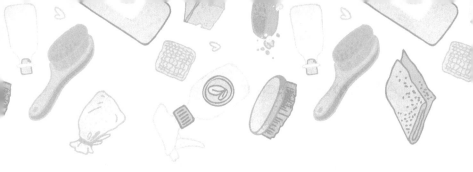

CHAPTER 11:
The Kitchen

I f you're like me, it probably feels like you spend more time in your kitchen than any other room in the house. Whether you're cooking a meal, packing the kids' lunches, eating dinner with the family, or cleaning up after a long day—chances are that you and your kitchen are very well acquainted.

That's why I like to start every Room-by-Room Analysis with the kitchen: because of its central role in our daily lives. The kitchen is universal; a symbol of family, togetherness, and love. It's the very heart of a home, and just like our hearts need care and attention to keep us strong and healthy, the same can be said about the heart of our home—the kitchen.

Product Spotlights

- All-Purpose Cleaner
- Cleaning Wipes
- Dish Soap
- Dishwasher Detergent
- Dishwasher Rinse Aid
- Disinfectant Spray
- Drain Cleaner
- Granite Cleaner
- Grout Cleaner
- Scrubbing Powder
- Oven Cleaner
- Plastic Containers

All-Purpose Cleaner

This simple cleaning spray is made with just two ingredients and will clean nearly every surface in your home. You can choose to add essential oils for a nice scent (about 10 drops), or you can do what I do and just use your favourite scent of castile soap.

Ingredients

- 2 cups (500 mL) distilled water
- 1 tablespoon (15 mL) castile soap
- Large spray bottle (at least 2 cups / 500 mL)

Directions

Add the water to the spray bottle, then add the castile soap. Cover the bottle and shake well before use.

Notes

Safe to use on all surfaces, including sealed stone and stainless steel.

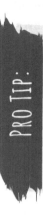

PRO TIP:

For stubborn messes or stuck-on grease, spray this all-purpose cleaner, followed by a generous sprinkle of baking soda. Let it sit for a few minutes, then scrub with a sponge and rinse. This tip works great for the stove and range hood where food messes and grease like to build up. For an even stronger cleaning spray, replace the castile soap with Sal Suds.

Alternative Options – All-Purpose Cleaner

Canada & USA

Aspen Clean	aspenclean.com
Attitude	attitudeliving.com
Better Life	cleanhappens.com
Biokleen	biokleenhome.com
Branch Basics	branchbasics.com
Clean Cult (LW)	cleancult.com
Common Good (LW)	commongoodandco.com
Counter Culture	countercultureclean.com
Dapple Baby	dapplebaby.com
Eco-Max	eco-max.com
Eco-Me	eco-me.com
ECOS	ecos.com
Ecostore	ecostoreusa.com
Fit Organic	fitorganic.com
Good Vibes (Black-owned)	goodvibesclean.com
GreenShield Organic	greenshieldorganic.com
Karmalades (Black-owned)	etsy.com/shop/karmalades
Koala Eco	koalaeco.com
Mama Suds	mamasuds.com
Meliora (LW)	meliorameansbetter.com
Murchison-Hume	murchison-hume.com
Nature Clean	natureclean.ca
Planet Luxe	wellbeingisland.com
Plant Therapy	planttherapy.com
PUR Home (Black-owned; LW)	shoppurhome.com
Saje Natural Wellness	saje.com
Sapadilla	sapadilla.com
Seventh Generation	seventhgeneration.com
Sun & Earth	sunandearth.com
The Green Laundress (Black-owned)	thegreenlaundress.com

Thieves	youngliving.com
Truce	truceclean.com
Whole Foods	wholefoodsmarket.com

Europe & UK

Elmkind (LW)	elmkind.co.uk
Greenscents	greenscents.co.uk
KINN	kinn-living.com
Mulieres (LW)	mulieres.eu
Murchison-Hume	murchison-hume.ch
Nu-Eco	nu-eco.co.uk
Ocean Saver (LW)	ocean-saver.com
Sonett	sonett.eu

Australia & New Zealand

Abode	healthyhomeproducts.com.au
EcoLogic	martinandpleasance.com/brands/ecologic
Ecostore	ecostore.com.au
EnviroCare Earth	envirocareearth.com.au
Ethique (LW)	ethique.com
Euclove	euclove.com.au
Herbon	herbon.com.au
Koala Eco	koala.eco
Koh (LW)	koh.com
Little Innoscents	littleinnoscents.com.au
Murchison-Hume	murchison-hume.com.au
OurEco Clean	ourecoclean.com.au
Planet Luxe	wellbeingisland.com.au
Resparkle (LW)	resparkle.com.au
Saba Organics	sabaorganics.com
Simply Clean (LW)	simplyclean.com.au
Sonett	sonett.com.au
The Botanical Life Co.	thebotanicallifeco.com.au

Africa

Better Earth	betterearth.co.za
Earthsap	faithful-to-nature.co.za/earthsap
Enchantrix	enchantrix.co.za
Mare & Itis	mareanditis.shop
Mrs. Martin's	mrsmartins.co.za
Natural Orange	faithful-to-nature.co.za/natural-orange
Nature Soap	naturesoap.co.za
Nu-Eco	nu-eco.co.za
Pure Simple (LW)	puresimple.co.za
Wellness Warehouse	wellnesswarehouse.com

Asia

Bio-home	biohomecares.com
Esona	esonaonline.com
Ethique (LW)	ethique.com
Gramp's	grampsasia.com
Pipper Standard	pippersingapore.com
Soapnut Republic	soapnutrepublic.com

Latin America

Biogar	biogar.co
Flor de Coco	flordecoco.mx
Newen	newen.mx
Pure & Sure	pureandsure.com.mx

Cleaning Wipes

These reusable cleaning wipes are inspired by the all-purpose cleaner in this chapter. They're more sustainable (and cheaper!) than disposable wipes since you can wash and reuse them over and over again.

Ingredients

- 1 ½ cups (375 mL) distilled water
- 1 tablespoon (15 mL) castile soap
- Small washcloths, or cut-up rags (20 to 30)
- Large glass jar with tight-fitting lid (a mason/pickle jar is perfect)

Directions

Add the water and soap to the container and stir. Add the cut-up cloths and press down to soak up all the solution. Cover the container and flip it upside down to ensure all the cloths are moistened.

To Use It

Pull out a cloth and squeeze out the excess liquid back in the jar. Wipe down your surfaces, then store used cloths in a small basket until laundry day.

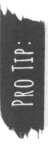 **PRO TIP:** Wash all cleaning cloths, microfibre towels, and kitchen towels on a hot water cycle, and use the Laundry Boosters in Chapter 13 to keep them fresh, clean, and disinfected.

Alternative Options – Cleaning Wipes

Canada & USA

All Clean Natural	allcleannatural.com
Aunt Fannie's	auntfannies.com
Babyganics	babyganics.com
Dapple Baby	dapplebaby.com
Elyptol	elyptol.com
Greenshield Organic	greenshieldorganic.com
Seventh Generation	seventhgeneration.com
Whole Foods	wholefoodsmarket.com

Dish Soap (Foam)

This simple foaming dish soap is inspired by the foaming hand soap recipe in the next chapter but uses Sal Suds—a gentle detergent—instead. Do not use castile soap in this recipe, it must be Sal Suds to work effectively.

Ingredients

- ¾ cup (180 mL) distilled water
- 2 tablespoons (30 mL) Sal Suds
- Foaming pump bottle

Directions

Add water to the foaming pump bottle first, then add Sal Suds. Cover and shake gently to combine.

Notes

Do not add this to a sink full of water—it will just dissipate without doing anything. Instead, use this for handwashing dishes by squirting the soap on a sponge and scrubbing dishes individually.

Alternative Options – Dish Soap (Foam)

Canada & USA

Attitude	attitudeliving.com
Fit Organic	fitorganic.com

Dish Soap (Liquid)

This liquid dish soap is great at cutting grease, and has a gel-like consistency, thanks to the kosher salt. Do not use castile soap in this recipe, it must be Sal Suds to work effectively.

Ingredients

- ½ cup (125 mL) distilled water, hot
- 2 teaspoons (10 g) kosher salt
- ½ cup (125mL) Sal Suds
- ½ cup (125 mL) white vinegar
- 1 teaspoon (5 g) citric acid
- Squeeze bottle or soap pump

Directions

In a small bowl, combine the hot water and kosher salt. Stir until dissolved, then set aside. In the squeeze bottle, add Sal Suds, vinegar, and citric acid, then swirl to combine. Add salt-water mixture to the squeeze bottle and gently shake until thickened.

Notes

Do not add this to a sink full of water—it will just dissipate without doing anything. Instead, use this for handwashing dishes by squirting the soap on a sponge and scrubbing dishes individually.

Alternative Options – Dish Soap (Liquid)

Canada & USA

Aspen Clean	aspenclean.com
Attitude	attitudeliving.com
Better Life	cleanhappens.com
Biokleen	biokleenhome.com
Clean Cult (LW)	cleancult.com
Common Good (LW)	commongoodandco.com
Dapple Baby	dapplebaby.com
Eco-Me	eco-me.com
ECOS	ecos.com
Ecostore	ecostoreusa.com
Ecover	ecover.com
Fit Organic	fitorganic.com
Green Cricket	greencricket.ca
Greenshield Organic	greenshieldorganic.com
Koala Eco	koalaeco.com
Made Of	madeof.com
Molly's Suds	mollyssuds.com
Murchison-Hume	murchison-hume.com
Nature Clean	natureclean.ca
Planet Luxe	wellbeingisland.com
Puracy	puracy.com
PUR Home (Black-owned; LW)	shoppurhome.com
Saje Natural Wellness	saje.com
Sapadilla	sapadilla.com
The Honest Co.	honest.com
Thieves	youngliving.com
Trader Joe's	traderjoes.com
Whole Foods	wholefoodsmarket.com
Yaya Maria's	yayamarias.com

Europe & UK

Ecover	ecover.com
Elmkind (LW)	elmkind.co.uk
Greenscents	greenscents.co.uk
Murchison-Hume	murchison-hume.ch
Nu-Eco	nu-eco.co.uk
Smol (LW)	smolproducts.com
Sodasan (sensitive)	sodasan.com
Sonett	sonett.eu

Australia & New Zealand

Abode	healthyhomeproducts.com.au
EcoLogic	martinandpleasance.com/brands/ecologic
Ecostore	ecostore.com.au
EnviroCare Earth	envirocareearth.com.au
Herbon	herbon.com.au
Kin Kin Naturals	kinkinnaturals.com.au
Koala Eco	koala.eco
Little Innoscents	littleinnoscents.com.au
Murchison-Hume	murchison-hume.com.au
Planet Luxe	wellbeingisland.com.au
Resparkle (LW)	resparkle.com.au
Saba Organics	sabaorganics.com
Simply Clean (LW)	simplyclean.com.au
Sonett	sonett.com.au

Africa

Better Earth	betterearth.co.za
Earthsap	faithful-to-nature.co.za/earthsap
Mrs. Martin's	mrsmartins.co.za
Natural Orange	faithful-to-nature.co.za/natural-orange
Nature Soap	naturesoap.co.za
Nu-Eco	nu-eco.co.za
Pure Simple (LW)	puresimple.co.za
Triple Orange	tripleorange.co.za

Asia

Arau	arau.jp
Bio-home	biohomecares.com
Gramp's	grampsasia.com
Miyoshi	miyoshisoap.co.jp
Pax Naturon	paxnaturon.com
Soapnut Republic	soapnutrepublic.com

Dishwasher Detergent (Liquid)

This liquid dishwasher detergent is made with Sal Suds and is boosted with the cleaning power of citric acid, vinegar, and lemons. The kosher salt helps thicken up this recipe to make it an easily pourable gel. Do not use castile soap in this recipe, it must be Sal Suds to work effectively.

Ingredients

- ½ cup (125 mL) white vinegar
- ½ cup (125 mL) distilled water, hot
- 1 tablespoon (20 g) kosher salt
- ½ cup (125 mL) Sal Suds
- 1 tablespoon (15 mL) lemon juice OR 10-15 drops lemon essential oil
- 3 tablespoons (45 g) citric acid powder
- Squeeze bottle (like a condiment bottle or upcycled dish soap bottle)

Directions

Add the vinegar to the squeeze bottle and set it aside. In a separate bowl, combine the hot water and kosher salt and stir to dissolve completely. Add the Sal Suds to the salt-water mixture and stir gently, then pour the solution into the squeeze bottle with the vinegar. Finally, add the lemon juice/essential oil and citric acid powder, cover the bottle, and shake well to combine.

To Use It

Add 1 tablespoon to the detergent compartment.

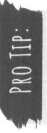

PRO TIP:

Natural dishwasher detergents (whether home-made or store-bought) will not be as strong and powerful as conventional ones. So give your dishes a quick soak/rinse to remove any stuck-on food bits before loading them in the dishwasher.

Alternative Options – Dishwasher Detergent (Liquid)

Canada & USA

Attitude	attitudeliving.com
Better Life	cleanhappens.com
Biokleen	biokleenhome.com
ECOS	ecos.com
Fit Organic	fitorganic.com
Mama Suds	mamasuds.com
Nature Clean	natureclean.ca
Puracy	puracy.com
The Honest Co.	honest.com
Whole Foods	wholefoodsmarket.com

Europe & UK

Sodasan	sodasan.com

Africa

Better Earth	betterearth.co.za
Earthsap	faithful-to-nature.co.za/earthsap
Triple Orange	tripleorange.co.za
Wellness Warehouse	wellnesswarehouse.com

Asia

Happy Elephant	happyelephant.jp

Dishwasher Detergent (Powder & Tabs)

This powdered dishwasher detergent recipe can be used as a loose powder or made into convenient grab-and-go tabs.

Ingredients

- 1 cup (240 g) washing soda
- 1 cup (200 g) borax
- ½ cup (160 g) kosher salt
- ½ cup (100 g) citric acid powder
- Large jar for storage
- Ice cube trays or silicone molds (if making tabs)

Directions

In a large bowl, slowly mix all the ingredients and add them to a large jar. Make sure not to mix too fast as it will create a dust cloud that you don't want to inhale. Alternately, you can add all ingredients to the jar first, then cover the jar and shake well to mix everything.

To use as a powder: Use 1 tablespoon per load. This mixture might clump or become solid over time. To prevent this, you can leave the mixture in the jar, uncovered, on the counter for a couple of days, making sure to stir it up gently several times a day. This helps release any moisture into the air. After a couple of days, you can cover the jar and store it.

To make tabs: Measure portions of about 1 tablespoon into the ice cube trays or silicone molds. Press with your thumb or the back of a spoon to firmly pack the mixture into the molds. Leave them out to dry on a counter for a couple of hours, then pop out the portions and store them in an airtight container. Use 1 tab per load.

Note

Washing soda is not the same as baking soda, and it is not safe for aluminum—so if you have aluminum pots and pans, or the inside of your dishwasher is lined with aluminum, try the liquid recipe on the previous page instead.

Alternative Options – Dishwasher Tabs

Canada & USA

Aspen Clean	aspenclean.com
Attitude	attitudeliving.com
Biokleen	biokleenhome.com
Blueland (LW)	blueland.com
Dapple	dapplebaby.com
Eco-Max	eco-max.com
ECOS	ecos.com
Ecostore	ecostoreusa.com
Mrs. Meyer's Clean Day	mrsmeyers.com
Nature Clean	natureclean.ca
Pardo Naturals (Black-owned)	pardonaturals.com
Puracy	puracy.com
Whole Foods	wholefoodsmarket.com

Europe & UK

Sonett	sonett.eu

Australia & New Zealand

Earthwise	earthwise.co.nz
Ecostore	ecostore.com.au
Lil'Bit	lilbit.com.au
Sonett	sonett.com.au

Alternative Options – Dishwasher Powder

Canada & USA

Biokleen	biokleenhome.com
Mama Suds	mamasuds.com
Nellie's	nelliesclean.com
Pardo Naturals (Black-owned)	pardonaturals.com

Europe & UK

Bio D	biod.co.uk
Nu-Eco	nu-eco.co.uk
Sonett	sonett.eu

Australia & New Zealand

Abode	healthyhomeproducts.com.au
EnviroCare Earth	envirocareearth.com.au
Herbon	herbon.com.au
Kin Kin Naturals	kinkinnaturals.com.au
Simply Clean (LW)	simplyclean.com.au
Sonett	sonett.com.au

Africa

Nu-Eco	nu-eco.co.za

Dishwasher Rinse Aid

This rinse aid is key to getting spotless dishes, especially if you're also using a homemade dishwasher detergent. It works to prevent hard water deposits and neutralizes the pH level of your water.

Ingredients

- ½ cup (125 mL) distilled water, hot
- 3 tablespoons (45 g) citric acid powder

Directions

Combine the hot water and citric acid in a bowl and stir until the powder is dissolved. Allow it to cool before pouring the mixture into the rinse aid compartment of your dishwasher.

Notes

Alternately, you can pour undiluted white vinegar into the rinse aid compartment; however, this may negatively affect the rubber seals in some newer dishwashers.

Alternative Options – Dishwasher Rinse Aid

Canada & USA

Eco-Max	eco-max.com
Eco-Me	eco-me.com
ECOS	ecos.com
Ecover	ecover.com
Nature Clean	natureclean.ca
The Honest Co.	honest.com

Europe & UK

Ecover	ecover.com
Sonett	sonett.eu

Australia & New Zealand

EnviroCare Earth	envirocareearth.com.au
Herbon	herbon.com.au
Sonett	sonett.com.au

Disinfectant Spray

Disinfect hard surfaces with this inexpensive and easy-to-use spray—it's made with just one ingredient!

Ingredients

- Hydrogen peroxide, 3%
- Old spray nozzle

Directions

Attach an old spray nozzle to a bottle of peroxide. After cleaning your surfaces, give them a quick spray of peroxide and let it air dry.

Why it works

Hydrogen peroxide is a stable and effective disinfectant when used on inanimate surfaces, and is active against a wide range of bacteria, viruses, and other microorganisms, according to the Centres for Disease Control.[39] It's safer than chlorine bleach, as it is odourless, colourless, and breaks down into just water and oxygen.

Notes

Peroxide must be stored in a dark bottle to stay active.

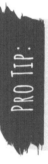

PRO TIP:

You can also disinfect your cutting boards after contact with raw meat. After washing your board to remove any bits of meat, spray the board with some peroxide, followed by a spray of white vinegar. Let it rest for 10-15 minutes, then rinse.

Alternative Options – Disinfectant Spray

Canada & USA

All Clean Natural (Wipes)	allcleannatural.com
Attitude	attitudeliving.com
PUR Home (Black-owned; LW)	shoppurhome.com
Seventh Generation	seventhgeneration.com
The Honest Co.	honest.com

Europe & UK

Nu-Eco	nu-eco.co.uk
Sodasan	sodasan.com

Australia & New Zealand

Earthwise	earthwise.co.nz
EnviroCare Earth	envirocareearth.com.au
Simply Clean (LW)	simplyclean.com.au
OurEco Clean	ourecoclean.com.au

Africa

Nu-Eco	nu-eco.co.za
So Pure	sopure.co.za

Drain Cleaner

Try this handy trick for attacking grease and fat that's slowing your kitchen drains. This method works better than the baking soda/vinegar trick that you may have tried in the past.

Ingredients

- ½ cup (140 g) table salt
- ½ gallon (2 litres) water, heated until almost boiling
- 1 teaspoon (5 mL) dish soap

Directions

Pour the salt down the drain. Add the dish soap to the hot water, then slowly pour the mixture down the drain. Flush with hot tap water.

Why It Works

This method attacks the grease that's clogging the pipes. The hot, soapy water melts the grease, and the salt helps scrub out the greasy build-up.

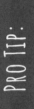

PRO TIP:

For maintenance, try using enzymatic drain sticks—small enzyme sticks that you drop into the drain, where they sit in the pipes, slowly releasing enzymes that break down grease and food. If you're dealing with a bathtub drain that's clogged with hair and soap scum, your best bet is to use a drain snake to pull out the clog. It's gross and unsightly, but it works. Both of these products can be found at any hardware store or online.

*I could not find a safer Alternative Option for this product.

Granite Cleaner

Clean your granite and natural stone counters and surfaces with this cleaning spray, specifically formulated to give those surfaces a beautiful shine. You can replace the castile soap with clear dish soap if that's all you have on hand.

Ingredients

- ¼ cup (60 mL) rubbing alcohol
- ½ tablespoon (7 mL) castile soap
- 10–20 drops essential oil (optional)
- 1 ½ cups (375 mL) distilled water

Directions

Add the alcohol, castile soap, and essential oils to a spray bottle and swirl to combine. Add the water and shake to mix well. Spray onto granite or any sealed stone surface, and wipe away with a microfibre cloth.

Notes

If the surface is still wet and won't dry, try buffing it with a dry cloth. You may also try increasing the alcohol to ½ cup (125 mL).

Alternative Options – Granite Cleaner

Canada & USA

Better Life	cleanhappens.com
Eco-Me	eco-me.com
Zum Clean	indigowild.com

Grout Cleaner

Clean and brighten your grout lines with this easy-to-use (and kind of fun!) grout cleaner. You'll be amazed by the results. You can replace the castile soap with clear dish soap if that's all you have on hand.

Ingredients

- ½ cup (115 g) baking soda
- ¼ cup (60 mL) hydrogen peroxide, 3%
- 1 teaspoon (5 mL) castile soap

Directions

Mix all the ingredients in a small bowl.

To use it

Apply the mixture onto grout lines with a small spoon. Wait 15 minutes, then scrub with an old toothbrush. Rinse with a wet cloth to remove excess cleaning mixture. Rinse the whole floor with a mop for a final rinse.

Notes

This mixture will expand and lose effectiveness over time; so only make what you will use in one session.

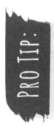 **PRO TIP:** For easier application, you can pour the mixture into a small squeeze bottle, and squeeze it directly onto the grout lines. This is a fun one to do with the kids!

*I could not find a safer Alternative Option for this product.

Scrubbing Powder

This is a dry powder scrubber, kind of like Comet, that you can use to scrub down your sinks when they get grimy. I like to keep a container of this by my kitchen sink so I can remember to use it every few days. It will give your sink a sparkling shine!

Ingredients

- 1 cup (230 g) baking soda
- ½ cup (140 g) table salt
- Dish soap
- Container with holes in the lid (upcycled spice jar, cheese shaker, etc.)

Directions

Mix baking soda and salt until combined, then store in a labelled container with holes in the lid.

To use it

Wet the surface and sprinkle the powder all over it. Add a small squirt of dish soap to a wet sponge, then scrub all surfaces. Rinse clean with water.

Notes

Safe to use on stainless steel and porcelain sinks. Do NOT use on stainless steel appliances. Use caution around acrylic or fibreglass surfaces. You can also add some borax or washing soda for extra cleaning action.

Alternative Options – Scrubbing Powder

Canada & USA

Aspen Clean	aspenclean.com
Bon Ami	bonami.com
Eco-Me	eco-me.com
PUR Home (Black-owned; LW)	shoppurhome.com
Truce	truceclean.com
Zum Clean	indigowild.com

Europe & UK

Sonett	sonett.eu

Australia

Sonett	sonett.com.au

Oven Cleaner

Tackle that dirty oven once and for all with this natural cleaner that won't stink up your kitchen with nasty fumes. It's a two-step process and may take longer (depending on how long it's been since it was last cleaned), but you'll just love your sparkling clean oven once it's done!

Ingredients

- ½ cup (115 g) baking soda
- 1 teaspoon (5 mL) castile soap
- 2 tablespoons (30 mL) water
- White vinegar in a spray bottle

Directions

Remove the oven racks. Combine the baking soda, castile soap, and water in a small bowl and mix to form a thick paste. Using your hands or a spoon, spread the paste all over the inside surfaces of the oven, including the door, glass, sides, and bottom (make sure to avoid the heating element!). Let the paste sit overnight for best results.

In the morning, spray all surfaces with the vinegar to create a foaming action. Using the rough side of a sponge, scrub all inside surfaces, focusing on any stubborn spots. You can also try using the side of a plastic card (like a credit card or gift card) to scrape off any stuck-on bits. Then, wipe with a wet cloth until rinsed clean and all residue is removed.

*I could not find a safer Alternative Option for this product.

Plastic Containers

Plastic has become a pervasive problem in society and it's very hard to remove it completely from our lives. If we understand the dangers it poses, we can make better decisions about what stays and what must go.

What's wrong with plastics?

Chemicals like Bisphenol-A (BPA) and phthalates have been found to leach into food and enter our bodies. According to a Yale University journal article,[40] BPA and phthalates have now been linked to "deformities of the male and female genitals, premature puberty in females, decreased sperm quality, and increases in breast and prostate cancers," among other health concerns.

Use these tips to reduce your exposure:
- Gradually bring more glass containers into your home (check thrift stores for second-hand pieces)
- Store leftovers in glass containers
- Replace plastic cooking utensils with wood or stainless steel alternatives
- Replace plastic water bottles with glass and stainless steel alternatives
- Use your plastic containers only for dry foods like sandwiches and snacks, and cold foods like fresh fruits and vegetables
- Repurpose old plastic containers to hold craft supplies, tools, office supplies, etc.
- Do not put plastics in the microwave or dishwasher (high heat breaks down plastics)

"

We dream of having a clean house
— but who dreams of actually
doing the cleaning?

— Marcus Buckingham

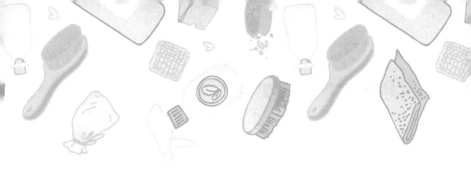

CHAPTER 12:

THE BATHROOM

I know, I know. Nobody likes cleaning the bathroom, and admittedly, it's the room that gets the least cleaning love from me. Instead of doing regular touch-ups like I'm supposed to, I leave it all to the last minute, which forces me to give it a deep cleaning every single time. This, of course, just makes me hate the job even more, and the whole cycle starts all over again.

But even if you're a bathroom cleaning Jedi Master who follows a meticulous schedule so the task never gets out of hand, chances are you don't particularly enjoy the smell of toxic bleach fumes slapping you in the face while you clean.

Most bathroom cleaning products contain bleach as the active ingredient, so they clean very well—a little too well—but you also have to deal with the strong odour during and after cleaning. So let's take care of that, shall we? Here are the specific products we'll focus on in the bathroom.

Product Spotlights

- All-Purpose Bathroom Cleaner
- Cleaning Scrub
- Daily Shower Spray
- Disinfectant Spray
- Hand Soap
- Hard Water Stain Remover
- Mould Remover
- Toilet Bowl Cleaner
- Shower Curtains

All-Purpose Bathroom Cleaner

This cleaning spray works great for all bathroom surfaces, including the toilet, floors, and counters. Just spray and wipe—and no toxic fumes!

Ingredients

- ½ teaspoon (3 g) washing soda
- ½ teaspoon (2 g) borax
- 1 tablespoon (15 mL) castile soap
- 2 cups (500 mL) warm water
- Large spray bottle

Directions

Add washing soda and borax to a spray bottle. Add warm water and swirl to dissolve the powders. Finally, add the soap, cover the bottle, and shake well to combine.

Notes

This cleaner does NOT contain a disinfectant. The simple Disinfectant Spray, found later in this chapter, can be sprayed on surfaces after using this cleaner.

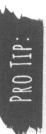

PRO TIP:

For sinks and tubs, you can spray this liberally, sprinkle baking soda all over, then scrub with a wet brush or sponge, and rinse clean. For tougher jobs, try the Cleaning Scrub in this chapter.

Alternative Options – Bathroom Cleaner

Canada & USA

Attitude	attitudeliving.com
Better Life	cleanhappens.com
Biokleen	biokleenhome.com
Common Good (LW)	commongoodandco.com
Eco-Max	eco-max.com
Eco-Me	eco-me.com
Ecostore	ecostoreusa.com
Ecover	ecover.com
Ethique (LW)	ethique.com
PUR Home (Black-owned; LW)	shoppurhome.com
Seventh Generation	seventhgeneration.com

Europe & UK

Ecover	ecover.com
Elmkind (LW)	elmkind.co.uk
Ethique (LW)	ethique.com
KINN	kinn-living.com
Nu-Eco	nu-eco.co.uk
Sodasan	sodasan.com
Sonett	sonett.eu

Australia & New Zealand

Abode	healthyhomeproducts.com.au
Earthwise	earthwise.co.nz
EcoLogic	martinandpleasance.com/ brands/ecologic
Ecostore	ecostore.com.au
EnviroCare Earth	envirocareearth.com.au
Ethique (LW)	ethique.com
Euclove	euclove.com.au
Green Potions	greenpotions.com.au
Koala Eco	koala.eco
Simply Clean (LW)	simplyclean.com.au
Sonett	sonett.com.au

Africa

Better Earth	betterearth.co.za
Earthsap	faithful-to-nature.co.za/ earthsap
Nu-Eco	nu-eco.co.za

Asia

Bio-home	biohomecares.com
Ethique (LW)	ethique.com
Pipper Standard	pippersingapore.com

Cleaning Scrub

This scrub easily cuts through soap scum and will brighten white surfaces. Use it to clean the bathtub, shower doors, tiles, and sinks.

Ingredients

- ¾ cup (175 g) baking soda
- ¼ cup (60 mL) castile soap
- 2 tablespoons (30 mL) hydrogen peroxide, 3% (optional, but helps whiten)

Directions

Add the baking soda and soap to a small bowl and stir well until you've made a paste. Add the peroxide and stir again. Apply to surfaces, scrub thoroughly with a brush or sponge, then rinse clean.

Notes

This scrub is best used right away but can be stored—without the peroxide—if needed. Store any leftover scrub in a sealed container.

Alternative Options – Cleaning Scrub

Canada & USA

Biokleen	biokleenhome.com
Eco-Me	eco-me.com
ECOS	ecos.com
Ecover	ecover.com
Meliora (LW)	meliorameansbetter.com
Pardo Naturals (Black-owned)	pardonaturals.com
The Green Laundress (Black-owned)	thegreenlaundress.com

Europe & UK

Ecover	ecover.com
Sodasan	sodasan.com
Sonett	sonett.eu

Australia & New Zealand

Green Potions	greenpotions.com.au
Lil'Bit	lilbit.com.au
OurEco Clean	ourecoclean.com.au
Sonett	sonett.com.au
The Botanical Life Co.	thebotanicallifeco.com.au

Africa

Cape of Storms	shopcapeofstorms.com
Earthsap	faithful-to-nature.co.za/earthsap
Natural Orange	faithful-to-nature.co.za/natural-orange

Asia

Soapnut Republic	soapnutrepublic.com

Daily Shower Spray

This shower spray is to be used between deep cleanings. It will prevent soap scum from forming, but it won't remove soap scum that's already there. For that, you'll need to use something like the Cleaning Scrub in this chapter.

Ingredients

- 1 cup (250 mL) distilled water
- ¼ cup (60 mL) hydrogen peroxide
- ¼ cup (60 mL) rubbing alcohol
- ½ teaspoon (3 mL) castile soap
- ½ tablespoon (7 mL) dishwasher rinse aid (optional)
- Spray bottle

Directions

Add all ingredients to a spray bottle and shake well. After each shower, while the surfaces are still wet, spray this all over the walls, curtain, shower doors, and fixtures. No need to rinse.

Notes

Peroxide breaks down when exposed to light, so use either a dark spray bottle, or wrap the bottle in a brown paper bag and always store it in a dark cupboard. Also, since the peroxide will degrade and lose its effectiveness over time, it's not recommended to make larger batches of this spray.

Alternative Options – Daily Shower Spray

Canada & USA

Attitude	attitudeliving.com
Better Life	cleanhappens.com
ECOS	ecos.com
Whole Foods	wholefoodsmarket.com

Disinfectant Spray

Disinfect hard surfaces with this inexpensive and easy-to-use spray—it's made with just one ingredient!

Ingredients

- Hydrogen peroxide, 3%
- Old spray nozzle

Directions

Attach an old spray nozzle to a bottle of peroxide. After cleaning your surfaces, give them a quick spray of peroxide and let it air dry.

Why it works

Hydrogen peroxide is a stable and effective disinfectant when used on inanimate surfaces, and is active against a wide range of bacteria, viruses, and other microorganisms, according to the Centres for Disease Control.[41] It's safer than chlorine bleach, as it is odourless, colourless, and breaks down into just water and oxygen.

Notes

Peroxide must be stored in a dark bottle to stay active.

Alternative Options – Disinfectant Spray

Canada & USA

Attitude	attitudeliving.com
PUR Home (Black-owned; LW)	shoppurhome.com
Seventh Generation	seventhgeneration.com
The Honest Co.	honest.com

Europe & UK

Nu-Eco	nu-eco.co.uk
Sodasan	sodasan.com

Australia & New Zealand

Earthwise	earthwise.co.nz
EnviroCare Earth	envirocareearth.com.au
Simply Clean (LW)	simplyclean.com.au
OurEco Clean	ourecoclean.com.au

Africa

Nu-Eco	nu-eco.co.za
So Pure	sopure.co.za

Hand Soap (Foam)

This is quite possibly the easiest product you could ever make. Just dilute some castile soap in water, and you're good to go.

Ingredients

- ¾ cup (180 mL) distilled water
- 2 tablespoons (30 mL) castile soap
- Foaming pump bottle (at least 1 cup/250 mL capacity)

Directions

Add water to the foaming pump bottle first, then add the soap and cover with the pump top. Gently shake to mix thoroughly, and it's ready to use!

Notes

These amounts are approximate. Just fill your bottle about 60% full with water and about 20% soap, leaving the rest of the space for the pump to fit without the liquid spilling over.

Alternative Options – Hand Soap (Foam)

Canada

Attitude	attitudeliving.com
Be Green Bath & Body	begreenbathandbody.com
Green Beaver	greenbeaver.com
Green Cricket	greencricket.ca
Hunnybunny (Black-owned)	hunnybunny.boutique
Kosmatology	kosmatology.com
Nature Clean	natureclean.ca
Pardo Naturals (Black-owned)	pardonaturals.com
Puracy	puracy.com
Rocky Mountain Soap Co.	rockymountainsoap.com
Saje Natural Wellness	saje.com
Sally B's Skin Yummies	sallybskinyummies.com
Southern Handmade Essentials (Black-owned)	shessentials17.com

Europe & UK

Sonett	sonett.eu

Australia & New Zealand

Resparkle (LW)	resparkle.com.au
Sonett	sonett.com.au

Asia

Arau	arau.jp
Pipper Standard	pippersingapore.com
Soapnut Republic	soapnutrepublic.com
Whamisa Organic Fruits	whamisa.com

Hand Soap (Liquid)

If you're looking for liquid soap, you can easily make some with grated/shredded bar soap and water. This one takes a little longer from start to finish, but you'll end up with a fairly large batch to last you a while.

Ingredients

- 2 cups (380 g) soap flakes (grated bar soap)
- 8 cups (2 litres) distilled water
- 2 tablespoons (30 mL) vegetable glycerin

Directions

Combine all the ingredients in a large pot. Cook over medium-low heat, stirring occasionally until the soap is dissolved, about 15 minutes. Let it cool for 12–24 hours, then transfer to jars, bottles, or other containers.

Notes

You can use this as hand soap and body wash. This soap will lather—not nearly as much as regular soap—but it still cleans!

Alternative Options – Hand Soap (Liquid)

Canada & USA

Alaffia	alaffia.com
All Clean Natural	allcleannatural.com
Attitude	attitudeliving.com
Aunt Fannie's	auntfannies.com
Dr. Bronner's	drbronner.com
ECOS	ecos.com
Hunnybunny (Black-owned)	hunnybunny.boutique
Karmalades (Black-owned)	etsy.com/shop/karmalades
Koala Eco	koalaeco.com
Mrs. Meyer's Clean Day	mrsmeyers.com
Nature Clean	natureclean.ca
Puracy	puracy.com
Rocky Mountain Soap Co.	rockymountainsoap.com
Seventh Generation	seventhgeneration.com
Soapply (LW)	soapplybox.com
Southern Handmade Essentials (Black-owned)	shessentials17.com
Yaya Maria's	yayamarias.com

Europe & UK

Conscious Skincare	conscious-skincare.com
Nu-Eco	nu-eco.co.uk
Sodasan	sodasan.com

Australia & New Zealand

Herbon	herbon.com.au
Koala Eco	koala.eco
Saba Organics	sabaorganics.com
Simply Clean (LW)	simplyclean.com.au

Africa

Earthsap	faithful-to-nature.co.za/earthsap
Enchantrix	enchantrix.co.za
Mrs. Martin's	mrsmartins.co.za
Nature Soap	naturesoap.co.za
Nu-Eco	nu-eco.co.za
Wellness Warehouse	wellnesswarehouse.com

Asia

Miyoshi	miyoshisoap.co.jp

Hard Water Stain Remover

Hard water deposits can be unsightly and quite difficult to remove, but this simple trick will have your fixtures sparkling in no time.

Ingredients

- White vinegar
- Small wash cloths/rags

Directions

Soak washcloths/rags in vinegar until completely saturated. Arrange or wrap the cloths around areas with hard water deposits (faucets, fixtures, drains, showerheads, etc.). Leave for at least an hour, adding more vinegar if needed to keep the cloths wet. Remove the cloths and clean the area with a clean towel.

Alternative Options – Hard Water Stains

Canada & USA

CLR	clrbrands.com
Fit Organic	fitorganic.com

Mould Remover

Zap away unsightly mould with this two-step process. The acidic vinegar and anti-fungal tea tree oil work together to kill the mould. Finish it off by scrubbing with peroxide to whiten the surface.

Ingredients

- ½ cup (125 mL) white vinegar
- 1 tablespoon (30 mL) tea tree oil
- Hydrogen peroxide, 3% (in a dark spray bottle)

Directions

Combine the vinegar and tea tree oil in a spray bottle, shake well, and spray it on mouldy surfaces. Allow the solution to sit for about 30 minutes to an hour without scrubbing. (Crack a window and turn on the fan, as the solution will smell very strong.) After 30 minutes, spray the area liberally with peroxide and scrub with an old toothbrush. Continue to spray and scrub several times until the surface is whitened, then wipe it clean with a microfiber cloth.

Notes

For mild cases and routine maintenance, one treatment should be enough. For severe cases, you may need to repeat the process a couple of times. To keep mould from coming back, you must identify the source of moisture; for example, always turn on the exhaust fan and crack a window while taking a shower.

Alternative Options – Mould Remover

Canada & USA

Concrobium Mold Control	concrobium.com

Europe & UK

Ecozone	ecozone.com

Australia & New Zealand

Abode	healthyhomeproducts.com.au
EnviroCare Earth	envirocareearth.com.au
OurEco Clean	ourecoclean.com.au
Simply Clean (LW)	simplyclean.com.au
Vrindavan	vrindavanbodycare.com

Africa

Pro-Nature	pronature.co.za

Toilet Bowl Cleaner Gel (Regular)

A simple toilet cleaner recipe that uses the cleaning power of soap, the scrubbing action of baking soda, and the disinfecting power of borax. Store this in a squeeze bottle to make it easy to apply to the inside of the bowl.

Ingredients

- 2 cups (500 mL) distilled water
- 1 cup (230 g) baking soda
- $^1/_3$ cup (70 g) borax (or more baking soda)
- $^1/_3$ cup (80 mL) castile soap
- 20 drops essential oils (optional)
- Squeeze bottle or upcycled condiment container

Directions

Mix the water, baking soda, and borax in a bowl until the powders dissolve. Funnel this mixture into an empty squeeze bottle. Slowly add the castile soap and essential oils to the bottle. Shake the container well to combine all ingredients. Use like any toilet cleaner gel—apply to the inside of toilet bowl, scrub, then flush.

Toilet Bowl Cleaner Gel (Extra Strength)

A more complex recipe that calls for a few specialty ingredients, this recipe is great for really tough cleaning jobs. It is also the closest thing you can get to making a commercial toilet cleaning gel at home.

Ingredients

- 1 teaspoon (3 g) xanthan gum
- 1 teaspoon (5 mL) vegetable glycerin
- 1 ½ cups (375 mL) hot water
- ½ cup (100 g) citric acid powder
- 25 drops essential oil (optional)
- Squeeze bottle or upcycled condiment container

Directions

In a bowl, mix the xanthan gum and glycerin and set them aside. In a separate bowl, mix the hot water and citric acid until it is completely dissolved. Add the xanthan gum solution to the citric acid solution and whisk well to combine. Pour it into a squeeze container. Let it cool and fully thicken for a few hours, then use it like any toilet cleaning gel—apply to the inside of toilet bowl, scrub, then flush.

Notes

The xanthan gum is used to thicken this cleaner so it will cling to the toilet bowl like the commercial cleaners. The glycerin is there to help the xanthan gum dissolve properly without clumping.

Toilet Bowl Cleaner (Spray)

The easiest of the 3 recipes, this toilet cleaner spray is great for quick cleanups. The borax is great for scrubbing and disinfecting, and it keeps the bowl cleaner for longer.

Ingredients

- All-Purpose Bathroom Cleaner (at the beginning of this chapter)
- Borax (stored in a jar with holes, like a cheese shaker)

Directions

Spray the inside of the toilet bowl with the All-Purpose Bathroom Cleaner in this chapter. Sprinkle borax in the toilet bowl, making sure to get it along the inside walls of the bowl as well. Scrub with a toilet brush, then flush.

Alternative Options – Toilet Bowl Cleaner

Canada & USA

Better Life	cleanhappens.com
Eco-Max	eco-max.com
Eco-Me	eco-me.com
ECOS	ecos.com
Ecostore	ecostoreusa.com
Ecover	ecover.com
Nature Clean	natureclean.ca

Europe & UK

Bio D	biod.co.uk
Ecover	ecover.com
Elmkind (LW)	elmkind.co.uk
Greenscents	greenscents.co.uk
Nu-Eco	nu-eco.co.uk
Sonett	sonett.eu

Australia & New Zealand

Abode	healthyhomeproducts.com.au
Earthwise	earthwise.co.nz
EcoLogic	martinandpleasance.com/brands/ecologic
Ecostore	ecostore.com.au
EnviroCare Earth	envirocareearth.com.au
Lil'Bit	lilbit.com.au
OurEco Clean	ourecoclean.com.au
Simply Clean (LW)	simplyclean.com.au
Sonett	sonett.com.au

Africa

Better Earth	betterearth.co.za
Earthsap	faithful-to-nature.co.za/earthsap
Enchantrix	enchantrix.co.za
Natural Orange	faithful-to-nature.co.za/natural-orange
Nu-Eco	nu-eco.co.za

Asia

Esona	esonaonline.com
Pax Naturon	paxnaturon.com
Soapnut Republic	soapnutrepublic.com

Shower Curtains

Most shower curtains and liners are made from a solid plastic called polyvinyl chloride (PVC), which is softened by the addition of phthalates. Shower curtains made with PVC can off-gas over 100 different volatile organic compounds into the air, according to a 2008 study that tested PVC shower curtains from five major US retailers.[42]

Why is PVC harmful?

As we've discussed in Chapters 1 and 5, VOCs and phthalates are linked to hormone disruption, asthma, certain types of cancer, and they contribute to indoor air pollution. Remember that "new curtain smell" after opening up a new shower curtain package? That's the smell of VOCs off-gassing into the air.

Alternative Options

The next time you're in the market for new shower curtains or liners, choose one of these safer, affordable options instead:

- **Polyester**: Quickest drying time; can be used as curtain or liner.
- **Nylon**: Dries quickly; can be used as curtain or liner.
- **Cotton**: Takes longer to dry; can develop mold, so should be used with a liner.
- **Linen**: Similar qualities to cotton.
- **Hemp**: Naturally resistant to bacteria; doesn't need a liner; dries quickly; more pricey.

LEVEL UP
YOUR JOURNEY!

We put together some amazing **Bonus Content** just for you! Visit **naturesnurtureblog.com/book** to access the complete library of bonus content that accompanies this book!

Here's what you'll get:

- Printables
- Direct Web Links
- Cheat Sheets
- Recipe Labels
- Checklists
- Reference Cards
- And more!

naturesnurtureblog.com/book

"

Behind every successful woman
is a basket of dirty laundry.

— SALLY FORTH

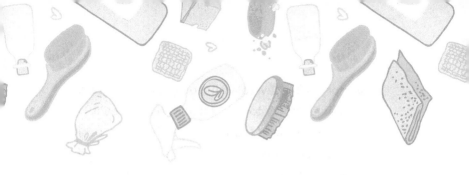

CHAPTER 13:
The Laundry Room

You would think the laundry room would be the cleanest in the house, but in fact, laundry products can be some of the most toxic products in your home.

Nearly all of the chemicals on The Worst Offenders list we looked at in Chapter 5 can be found in laundry products. So if someone in your home has sensitive skin, allergies, or asthma, chances are your conventional laundry products aren't helping. But before we jump right into the recipes and product recommendations, there are a few things we need to discuss first.

Ditch the Fabric Softeners

Even if you're happy with your laundry detergent and don't see a need to replace it, my second recommendation is to try and ditch the fabric softener. I know, this one sounds hard because who doesn't want soft laundry? But I promise it's worth it. And once you've detoxed your laundry routine, you won't even miss the fabric softeners.

True story: After several visits to my mom's house and dealing with stinky towels, I finally discovered it was her beloved bottle of fabric softener that was causing the awful sour smell that seemed to be embedded in her towels and linens. I had recently convinced her to switch to a natural detergent, but apparently, she was still using the fabric softener with every load. And boy, was it noticeable!

Once we stripped those towels and linens with the Laundry Stripping Solution described in this chapter, the smell was completely gone, and everything was so clean and fresh. Needless to say, I made her throw out the last of her fabric softener and promise never to buy it again. Problem solved!

Trust me. Ditch your fabric softener—you'll thank me later. Then use the DIY recipe included in this chapter.

Stripping Your Laundry

Remember when we discussed QACs and Optical Brighteners and how they're designed to stay on your fabrics—even after they've been rinsed out with water? As it turns out, those chemicals accumulate over time and can leave behind a funky buildup on your laundry. As long as you're using mainstream laundry detergents, you may not even notice this buildup. But once you make the switch to more natural products, the buildup becomes more evident.

So before you switch over to a natural detergent, I highly recommend you "strip" your laundry first, to remove any of that buildup left behind from years of conventional laundry products. Otherwise, you might end up with stinky laundry because the natural detergent won't be able (and wasn't designed) to remove all that leftover gunk.

To learn how to do this, simply follow the instructions in this chapter under the "Laundry Stripping Solution" section.

Homemade Laundry Soap

There's no shortage of recipes online for homemade laundry soaps, made with various ingredients, that are indeed better for your health than the conventional stuff you buy at the store. In fact, laundry soap was one of the very first products I made at home when I started my non-toxic journey. The original recipe is still posted on my blog, and I used it for many, many years before I ultimately decided to stop—and I'll tell you why.

This will probably ruffle some feathers since it's a bit controversial, but I've written about this on the blog already,[43] so I'll share it here as well.

To make a long story short, I no longer use homemade laundry soaps because I've found that the soap in these recipes has a hard time dissolving properly in the wash water, and an even harder time rinsing away completely without leaving behind a residue (i.e. soap scum) that can build up in your fabrics over time.

Now there are several factors involved that could make this true/untrue for your specific situation, and in fact, many people continue to use these recipes with great results. Water temperature, water hardness, fabric type, machine type—all of these can drastically change your results with homemade laundry soaps, so your results may vary.

But in the spirit of supporting you in choosing your own path on this journey, I've included my original recipes for both powder and liquid laundry soap in this chapter. I will say that if you have soft water, you'll have much better results with them than if you have hard water. If you do choose to use one of these recipes, I highly recommend that you also use the DIY fabric softener, since it will help remove the soap scum that could be left behind on your clothes.

I also encourage you to read the post on my blog in which I delve much deeper into this topic—you can access the post directly at this link: bit.ly/DIYSoapProblem

Product Spotlights

- Laundry Stripping Solution
- Dryer Sheets
- Fabric Softener
- Laundry Boosters & Bleach Alternatives
- Laundry Detergent
- Stain Pre-soak Solution
- Stain Remover & Pre-treater

Laundry Stripping Solution

Ingredients

- 1 cup (230 g) baking soda
- 1 cup (240 g) washing soda
- 1 cup (200 g) borax
- 1 tablespoon (15 mL) Sal Suds (or one small scoop/ measure of natural detergent)

Directions

Add all the ingredients to the washing machine. Set the machine to a HOT water cycle and let it fill with water. Stir the powders to dissolve them in the water, then add your laundry. Leave the lid open and let the laundry soak for four hours, or until the water cools. Then close the lid and let the machine complete the cycle. This method is for use in a top-loader machine. For front-loaders, please see alternate instructions below.

Notes

If your machine won't allow you to delay the cycle to let the laundry soak, you can just run the cycle as normal and still get results. The soaking time does increase the cleaning power, but the solution will still work without the soak.

For front-loaders: Alternately, if you don't have a top loader machine, you can use a large bucket or your bathtub for this process; simply fill the tub about halfway with HOT water, dissolve the powders and soap, add the laundry, and let it soak for four hours. Then wring out excess water from laundry, place it in the washing machine, and run a wash cycle with water only.

Warning

Washing soda should not be used on aluminum surfaces, so if your washing machine is made of aluminum on the inside, do not include the washing soda in this stripping solution.

Alternative Options – Laundry Stripping Solution

Canada & USA

GroVia Mighty Bubbles	grovia.com
RLR Laundry Treatment	

Dryer Sheets

These reusable sheets will scent your laundry without the overpowering smell of artificial fragrances or the film that commercial sheets leave behind on your clothes.

Ingredients

- Small piece of cotton cloth (about 6–8 inches)
- 5 drops essential oil (orange or lavender is great)

Directions

Soak the cotton cloth with water and wring it out so it's just damp. Add about five drops of your favourite essential oil all over the cloth. Throw the cloth into the dryer along with your laundry. Just keep rewetting the cloth and using it for each load until the smell runs out. Then toss it in the wash and start all over again.

Notes

This works best if it's done in the last 10 minutes of drying. Or you may choose to run a quick, no-heat cycle with the dryer sheet after the main drying cycle is complete.

Wool Dryer Balls

Another option—my favourite!—is placing some wool dryer balls in the dryer. These balls help fluff up laundry and reduce static and overall drying time. You can also add a few drops of essential oil to each ball for a nice scent.

PRO TIP: To help reduce static, attach a safety pin to the dryer balls.

Alternative Options – Dryer Sheets

Canada & USA

Attitude Reusable Cloths	attitudeliving.com
PurEcosheet Reusable Dryer Sheets	purecosheet.com

Global

Wool Dryer Balls (various brands)

Fabric Softener

This simple mixture will soften your laundry and rinse away any remaining detergent or residue from your clothes.

Ingredients

- 1 gallon (4 litres) distilled water, warm (or tap water, boiled and cooled)
- 1 cup (200 g) citric acid powder
- Large container with pourable spout

Directions

Add water and citric acid to a large container. Cover and shake well until the powder dissolves.

To use it

Add ½ cup (125 mL) softener solution in the rinse cycle of your washer. If you have a fabric softener dispenser, you can add it there. Or use a fabric softener ball to automatically dispense it during the rinse cycle.

Notes

Alternately, you can pour about ½ cup (125 mL) undiluted white vinegar into the rinse aid compartment; however, this may negatively affect the rubber seals in some newer washing machines (older machines seem to be fine).

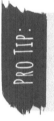
PRO TIP: If you're using a homemade laundry soap, you want to make sure to use either the vinegar or citric acid solution in the fabric softener compartment. It helps remove any buildup that might be left behind.

I highly advise against the use of commercial fabric softeners, so there are no Alternative Options for this product.

Laundry Boosters & Bleach Alternatives

Use any of the following ingredients to help boost your laundry and keep it looking and feeling its best. You can use just one or a combination, depending on what you're looking to achieve.

Ingredients

- ½ cup (115 g) baking soda
  (freshener, brightener, odour remover)
- ½ cup (120 g) washing soda
  (stain fighter, water softener)
- ½ cup (100 g) borax
  (whitener, water softener, odour remover, disinfectant)
- ½ cup (125 mL) hydrogen peroxide
  (whitener and brightener)

Directions

Add ½ cup of any one (or a combination) of these ingredients to your washer as it's filling up with water—*before* you add your laundry. The peroxide can go right into your machine's bleach dispenser if it has one. If you're using cold water to wash, you may need to dissolve the powders (the sodas and borax) in a separate cup of warm water first, then add them to the washing machine.

Notes

For **front-loader machines,** use half the amounts listed above. Sprinkle the powder boosters in the empty washer drum before adding laundry, and add the peroxide to the bleach compartment in your machine.

PRO TIP:

My default—especially for the kids' clothes, kitchen towels, and my workout clothes—is a combination of washing soda and borax.

Alternative Options – Laundry Boosters & Bleach Alternatives

Canada & USA

Biokleen	biokleenhome.com
Eco-Me	eco-me.com
Ecover	ecover.com
Oxi Clean (Baby or Free version)	oxiclean.com
ECOS OXO Brite	ecos.com
Molly's Suds	mollyssuds.com
Nature Clean	natureclean.ca
Nellie's	nelliesclean.com
PUR Home (Black-owned; LW)	shoppurhome.com
Seventh Generation	seventhgeneration.com
Simply Clean	simply-clean.ca
The Soap Works	puresoapworks.com

Europe & UK

Bio D	biod.co.uk
Ecover	ecover.com
Nu-Eco	nu-eco.co.uk
Sodasan	sodasan.com
Sonett	sonett.eu

Australia & New Zealand

Earthwise	earthwise.co.nz
Mi Eco	mieco.com.au
Sonett	sonett.com.au

Africa

Nature Soap	naturesoap.co.za
Nu-Eco	nu-eco.co.za
The Apothecary	theapothecary.co.za

Asia

Arau	arau.jp
Soapnut Republic	soapnutrepublic.com

Latin America

Flor de Coco	flordecoco.mx

Laundry Detergent (Liquid)

As mentioned in the introduction to this chapter, this soap-based laundry liquid might leave a buildup on your laundry and/or washer. I share the recipe here because some people do love it. Again, it's recommended to also use the homemade fabric softener recipe in this chapter to help reduce any soap scum buildup.

Ingredients

- 1 cup (240 g) washing soda
- ½ cup (125 g) kosher salt
- 1 cup (200 g) borax (optional)
- 1 cup (250 mL) liquid castile soap
- 1 gallon (4 litres) hot water, divided
- 2-gallon bucket with a lid (from the hardware store)

Directions

In the 2-gallon bucket, add ½ gallon (2 litres) of hot water, plus the washing soda, salt, and borax, and stir well to dissolve. In a large bowl, mix 4 cups (1 litre) of hot water with the castile soap and stir well. Add the soap/water mixture to the washing soda/borax/salt mixture in the bucket. Pour slowly and stir as you pour. Add 4 cups (1 litre) of hot water, and stir again. Let the soap cool, stirring occasionally. It may thicken up and gel, or it may separate—use a whisk or stick blender to get it to a smooth consistency.

To use it

Top-loader: Add ½ cup (125 mL) to detergent dispenser.

Front-loader: Add 2 to 3 tablespoons (30 mL to 45 mL) to detergent dispenser.

PRO TIP: Add about ½ cup (125 mL) white vinegar to the rinse cycle (or into the fabric softener compartment in your machine). Or you can make the homemade fabric softener solution mentioned earlier in this chapter.

Alternative Options – Laundry Liquid

Canada & USA

Aspen Clean	aspenclean.com
Attitude	attitudeliving.com
Babyganics	babyganics.com
Better Life	cleanhappens.com
Common Good (LW)	commongoodandco.com
Dapple Baby	dapplebaby.com
Eco-Max	eco-max.com
Eco-Me	eco-me.com
Fit Organic	fitorganic.com
Greenshield Organic	greenshieldorganic.com
Molly's Suds	mollyssuds.com
Murchison-Hume	murchison-hume.com
Nature Clean	natureclean.ca
Planet Luxe	wellbeingisland.com
Pure Natural	purenaturalcleaners.com
PUR Home (Black-owned; LW)	shoppurhome.com
Sapadilla	sapadilla.com
Thieves	youngliving.com

Europe & UK

Bio D	biod.co.uk
Greenscents	greenscents.co.uk
Mulieres (LW)	mulieres.eu
Murchison-Hume	murchison-hume.ch
Nu-Eco	nu-eco.co.uk
Ocean Saver (LW)	ocean-saver.com
Smol (LW)	smolproducts.com
Sonett (sensitive version)	sonett.eu

Australia & New Zealand

Abode	healthyhomeproducts.com.au
EcoLogic	martinandpleasance.com/brands/ecologic
EnviroCare Earth	envirocareearth.com.au
Herbon	herbon.com.au
Kin Kin Naturals	kinkinnaturals.com.au
Koala Eco	koala.eco
Little Innoscents	littleinnoscents.com.au
Murchison-Hume	murchison-hume.com.au
Planet Luxe	wellbeingisland.com.au
Saba Organics	sabaorganics.com
Simply Clean (LW)	simplyclean.com.au
Sonett (sensitive)	sonett.com.au

Africa

Better Earth	betterearth.co.za
Earthsap	faithful-to-nature.co.za/earthsap
Enchantrix	enchantrix.co.za
Mrs. Martin's	mrsmartins.co.za
Nu-Eco	nu-eco.co.za
Pure Simple (LW)	puresimple.co.za
Wellness Warehouse	wellnesswarehouse.com

Asia

Arau	arau.jp
Bio-home	biohomecares.com
Esona	esonaonline.com
Miyoshi	miyoshisoap.co.jp
Pax Naturon	paxnaturon.com
Pipper Standard	pippersingapore.com
Soapnut Republic	soapnutrepublic.com

Latin America

Biogar	biogar.co
Nama	nama.mx
Newen	newen.mx

Laundry Detergent (Powder)

As mentioned in the introduction to this chapter, this soap-based laundry powder might leave a buildup on your laundry and/or washer. I share the recipe here because some people do love it. If washing in cold water, you may need to dissolve the soap mixture in warm/hot water first before adding it to your machine.

Ingredients

- 1 cup (190 g) finely grated bar soap
- 2 cups (200 g) borax (or 2 cups / 450 g baking soda)
- 2 cups (480 g) washing soda
- ½ cup (125 g) kosher salt

Directions

Add all the ingredients to a large bowl. Slowly mix everything, being careful not to inhale any of the dust. Store it in an airtight container.

To Use It

Top-loader: Add 3 to 4 tablespoons (45 to 60 g) to detergent dispenser.

Front-loader: Add 1 to 2 tablespoons (15 to 30 g) to detergent dispenser.

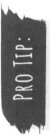

PRO TIP: Add about ½ cup (125 mL) white vinegar to the rinse cycle (or into the fabric softener compartment in your machine). Or you can make the homemade fabric softener solution mentioned earlier in this chapter.

Alternative Options – Laundry Powder

Canada & USA

Molly's Suds	mollyssuds.com
Nature Clean	natureclean.ca
Pardo Naturals (Black-owned)	pardonaturals.com
PUR Home (Black-owned; LW)	shoppurhome.com
The Green Laundress (Black-owned)	thegreenlaundress.com
The Soap Works	puresoapworks.com
TruEarth Strips (LW)	tru.earth

Europe & UK

Bio D	biod.co.uk
Sonett	sonett.eu

Australia & New Zealand

Abode	healthyhomeproducts.com.au
Earthwise	earthwise.co.nz
EnviroCare Earth	envirocareearth.com.au
Green Potions	greenpotions.com.au
Herbon	herbon.com.au
Lil'Bit	lilbit.com.au
Resparkle (LW)	resparkle.com.au
Sonett	sonett.com.au

Africa

Cape of Storms	shopcapeofstorms.com
Earthsap	faithful-to-nature.co.za/earthsap
Natural Orange	faithful-to-nature.co.za/natural-orange
Nature Soap	naturesoap.co.za

Asia

Happy Elephant	happyelephant.jp
Miyoshi	miyoshisoap.co.jp
Soapnut Republic	soapnutrepublic.com

Latin America

Flor de Coco	flordecoco.mx

Stain Pre-Soak Solution

When you need a tough solution to get stubborn stains out of your laundry, this pre-soak is very effective, thanks to the combination of peroxide and washing soda. This works great on kids' clothes to remove grass, marker, and food stains.

Ingredients

- 2 gallons (8 litres) warm water
- 1 cup (250 mL) hydrogen peroxide
- ½ cup (120 g) washing soda
- Large bucket/tub

Directions

Pour the warm water into the bucket. Add the peroxide and washing soda and stir to dissolve. Soak the clothing item(s) in the solution for at least 3–4 hours, making sure to stir/agitate it every hour or so. Wash the item(s) in the washer as usual, and discard the soaking solution (you can pour it down the drain).

Notes

This solution is safe to use on coloured fabric as long as the peroxide is diluted in the water *before* the clothing items are put into the solution. If you're still worried about discolouration, try one of the Alternative Options for Laundry Boosters or Stain Removers on previous page.

Stain Remover & Pre-Treater

This pre-treater works best if you use it while the stain is still fresh (up to a day or two). For more set-in stains, try the Pre-Soak Solution in this chapter.

Ingredients

- ½ cup (125 mL) hydrogen peroxide
- ¼ cup (60 mL) Sal Suds (or clear dish soap)
- Baking soda
- Small, dark spray bottle

Directions

Add the peroxide and soap to the dark spray bottle.

To Use It

Sprinkle some baking soda on the stain. Shake the peroxide/soap mixture and spray it over the baking soda until it is saturated. Rub the stain with a toothbrush. Let it sit for at least 10 minutes, then wash as usual.

Notes

May not be safe for some colour fabrics. Do a spot test in a hidden area if you're not sure. Or use one of the Alternative Options below. As with any stain, make sure the stain is gone before putting the item in the dryer! Otherwise, the dryer heat will set the stain, making it much more difficult to remove.

Alternative Options – Stain Remover

Canada & USA

All Clean Natural	allcleannatural.com
Attitude	attitudeliving.com
Babyganics	babyganics.com
Better Life	cleanhappens.com
Biokleen Bac Out	biokleenhome.com
ECOS	ecos.com
Ethique (LW)	ethique.com
Fit Organic	fitorganic.com
Meliora (LW)	meliorameansbetter.com
Molly's Suds	mollyssuds.com
Murchison-Hume	murchison-hume.com
Nature Clean	natureclean.ca
Nellie's	nelliesclean.com
Simply Clean	simply-clean.ca
The Soap Works	puresoapworks.com

Europe & UK

Ecoleaf	suma.coop
Ethique (LW)	ethique.com
Sodasan	sodasan.com

Australia & New Zealand

EcoLogic	martinandpleasance.com/brands/ecologic
EnviroCare Earth	envirocareearth.com.au
Ethique (LW)	ethique.com
Green Potions	greenpotions.com.au
Herbon	herbon.com.au
Kin Kin Naturals	kinkinnaturals.com.au
Murchison-Hume	murchison-hume.com.au

Africa

Pure Simple (LW)	puresimple.co.za

Asia

Ethique (LW)	ethique.com
Gramp's	grampsasia.com
Miyoshi	miyoshisoap.co.jp
Pipper Standard	pippersingapore.com

Enjoying the Book So Far?

The BEST way to thank an author is to post a review online.

If you're enjoying this book, would you please leave a review on **Amazon** or **Goodreads**? It would be greatly appreciated. Thank you!

And you can always reach me by email if you'd like to chat: sarah@naturesnurtureblog.com

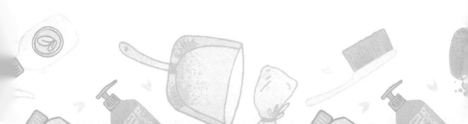

"

The first step in crafting the
life you want is to get rid of
everything you don't.

— JOSHUA BECKER

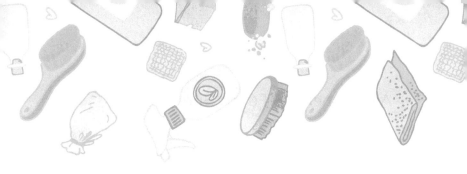

CHAPTER 14:

THE LIVING AREAS

I n this chapter, we're going to focus on products that are commonly used all over the home, not necessarily in one specific space. Besides the floors and windows, I want you to pay close attention to the section on air fresheners. Because we want to avoid artificial fragrances and other dangerous chemicals in the air, I would argue this is one of the most important sections you will read in this analysis.

Product Spotlights

- Air Freshener
  & Fabric Spray
- Air Freshener Options
- Air Purifying
  Indoor Plants
- Carpet & Mattress
  Deodorizer
- Carpet Shampoo
  (for machines)
- Carpet Stain Remover
- Floor Cleaners
- Glass & Window Cleaner
- Pest Control Spray
- Wood Furniture Polish

Air Freshener & Fabric Spray

Freshen up your room, linens, and furniture with a light scent, using safer ingredients and natural fragrance from essential oils.

Ingredients

- 2 tablespoons (30 mL) witch hazel (or rubbing alcohol)
- 10–20 drops essential oil
- ½ cup (125 mL) distilled water
- Small fine-mist spray bottle

Directions

Add the witch hazel (or rubbing alcohol) and essential oils to the spray bottle. Swirl the bottle about 10 times to combine oils with witch hazel. Top off with water, leaving a little room at the top for shaking.

Notes

Do not spray directly on fabrics, as the oils may leave spots on furniture. Instead, spray it high above in the air, allowing it to slowly settle down on the fabric. As with all products containing essential oils, use caution around children and pets. See Safety Info in the Appendix at the end of this book.

Alternative Options – Air Freshener & Fabric Spray

Canada & US

Aura Cacia	auracacia.com
Counter Culture	countercultureclean.com
Eco-Max	eco-max.com
Eco-Me	eco-me.com
ECOS	ecos.com
Grow Fragrance (My favourite)	growfragrance.com
Homeocan Essencia	homeocan.ca
Karmalades (Black-owned)	etsy.com/shop/karmalades
Koala Eco	koalaeco.com
Pardo Naturals (Black-owned)	pardonaturals.com
Plant Therapy	planttherapy.com
Saje Natural Wellness	saje.com
Southern Handmade Essentials (Black-owned)	shessentials17.com
Truce	truceclean.com
Zum Clean	indigowild.com

Europe & UK

Nu-Eco	nu-eco.co.uk

Australia & New Zealand

Earthwise	earthwise.co.nz
Euclove	euclove.com.au
Koala Eco	koala.eco
Lemon Myrtle Fragrances	lemonmyrtlefragrances.com.au
Lil'Bit	lilbit.com.au
OurEco Clean	ourecoclean.com.au
The Botanical Life Co.	thebotanicallifeco.com.au

Africa

Better Earth	betterearth.co.za
Mrs. Martin's	mrsmartins.co.za
Nu-Eco	nu-eco.co.za
Wellness Warehouse	wellnesswarehouse.com

Asia

Gramp's	grampsasia.com

Other Air Freshener Options

Aside from room and fabric sprays, here are some other options for freshening your home while also creating a nice atmosphere.

Ultrasonic Diffusers

Diffusers use tap water and essential oils (but distilled water is preferred). They work by sending tiny, ultrasonic vibrations into the water, which then break down the essential oils into micro molecules and projects (diffuses) them into the air. They are especially great during cold/flu season, and can also act as a cool-mist humidifier during the dry winter months.

You can find diffusers at most home goods stores or online retailers. Make sure the essential oils you use are of the highest quality you can find and only contain 100% essential oils (no fragrance oils). A list of trusted essential oils brands is available in the Appendix.

Candles

Most candles are made from paraffin wax, a petroleum byproduct that releases black soot and toxic chemicals into the air—many of which are known carcinogens (cancer causers) and can aggravate conditions like asthma and heart problems.

Safer options include beeswax, coconut wax, or soy wax candles. Make sure they are scented with 100% essential oils to avoid the harmful effects of synthetic fragrances. Non-toxic candles can be a little difficult to find in stores, so you may have to resort to online options.

Alternative Options – Candles

Canada & USA

Bee Hive Candles	beehivecandles.com
Cellar Door	cellardoorcandles.com
Dani Naturals	daninaturals.com
Fontana Candle Co.	fontanacandlecompany.com
Grow Fragrance	growfragrance.com
Lohn	shoplohn.com
Nashville Wax Co.	nashvillewaxco.com
Natural Annie Essentials (Black-owned)	naturalannieessentials.com
Pure Plant Home	pureplanthome.com
Slow North	slownorth.com
Terralite	terralite.com
The Good Soy	thegoodsoy.com
UMA	umaoils.com
Woodlot	shopwoodlot.ca

Europe & UK

AromaWorks	aroma-works.com
Bolt & Star	boltandstar.com
Eym	eymnaturals.com
Irusu	irusu.co.uk
Lola's Apothecary	lolasapothecary.com

Australia & New Zealand

Celia Loves	celialoves.com.au
ECO Modern Essentials	ecomodernessentials.com.au
Lemon Canary	lemoncanary.com.au
Northern Light Candle Company	northernlightscandles.com
Queen B	queenb.com.au
Salus	salusbody.com.au
Willows Scentials	willowscandles.com.au

Asia

BeCandle	becandle.com.hk
Essencial Candles	essencialcandles.com
Moonglade Candle	moongladecandle.com
MYBU Candles	mybucandle.com

Air Purifying Houseplants

A great way to improve the air quality in your home is to add some indoor plants! Not only do they look beautiful, but house plants can also clean and filter indoor air to remove toxins, as well as reduce mould spores and bacteria.

The Science

In 1989, scientists at NASA conducted a Clean Air Study and identified 12 houseplants that remove (or reduce) indoor air pollutants and gases, like benzene and formaldehyde, among others.[44] For more than 30 years, the lead scientist for that study, Dr. B.C. Wolverton, has produced some of the most well-known and reputable research papers on this topic.

He also published a book, *How to Grow Fresh Air: 50 Houseplants that Purify Your Home and Office*, which explains more of his findings and ranks the plants in descending order from the most effective at removing air pollutants, to the least. Each plant has its own two-page spread with a full-colour photo, information on how to care for the plant, and which specific toxins it removes from the air. If you're looking to bring more houseplants into your home and need some guidance, I highly recommend this book!

I've compiled 15 of my favourite plants from Dr. Wolverton's book into a chart on the next page. They're listed in the same order that they appear in the book—from the most effective to the least—and their scientific names are provided in parenthesis. These are plants that I've grown myself and are fairly easy to find at your local garden centre.

The only thing missing from the book, that I wish he would have included, is a warning about the possible toxicity of each plant. Most houseplants are toxic if ingested and can cause mild to severe reactions, so it's important to keep them out of reach of small children and pets. I've added a column in the chart to indicate whether or not each plant is safe to keep around pets, according to the American Society for the Prevention of Cruelty to Animals (ASPCA) website.[45]

List of Plants

1. Bamboo/Parlor Palm (*Chamaedorea seifrizii*)   SAFE
2. Rubber Plant (*Ficus robusta*)   NOT
3. Dracaena "Janet Craig" (*Dracaena dermensis*)   NOT
4. Dwarf Date Palm (*Phoenix roebelenii*)   SAFE
5. Boston Fern (*Nephrolepis exaltata "Bostoniensis"*)   SAFE
6. Peace Lily (*Spathiphyllum*)   NOT
7. Golden Pothos (*Epipremnum aureum*)   NOT
8. Gerbera Daisy (*Gerbera jamesonii*)   SAFE
9. Dragon Tree (*Dracaena marginata*)   NOT
10. Dumb Cane (*Dieffenbachia camilla*)   NOT
11. Snake Plant (*Sansevieria trifasciata / laurentii*)   NOT
12. Prayer Plant (*Maranta leuconeura "Kerchoveann"*)   SAFE
13. Dwarf Banana (*Musa cavendishii*)   SAFE
14. Spider Plant (*Chlorophytum comosum*)   SAFE
15. Moth Orchid (*Phalaenopsis*)   SAFE

Carpet & Mattress Refresher

Freshen up your carpets, mattresses, pet bedding, and more with this quick and easy deodorizer made with just baking soda and essential oils.

Ingredients

- 1 cup (230 g) baking soda
- 10-15 drops essential oil (optional; omit if you have pets)
- Container with holes in lid (spice jar, cheese shaker, etc.)

Directions

Add the baking soda to the container. Add the essential oils, then stir to distribute the oils evenly. Cover the container.

To use it

Sprinkle the powder over carpets, mattresses, or other furniture. Let sit for 10–30 minutes, then vacuum thoroughly.

Notes

If you have pets, leave out the essential oils and just use plain baking soda.

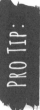

PRO TIP: If you don't have a container with holes in the lid, you can try using a kitchen sifter to sift the mixture onto the surfaces you want to freshen up.

Carpet Shampoo (For Machines)

Use this simple solution in your carpet cleaning machine to remove stains and deep clean your carpets.

Ingredients

- Hot water
- 2–3 drops Sal Suds (or clear dish soap)

Directions

Fill the carpet cleaner tank with hot water, then add the Sal Suds. Clean your carpets with the machine, making sure to properly rinse the solution out of your carpet (according to the manufacturer's instructions).

Before using the machine

Pre-treat tough stains first with the All-Purpose Cleaner in Chapter 11. Simply spray on stains and rub it in with your fingers or a small brush. Then proceed with using the machine as normal.

Warning

Make sure that using a solution like this won't void your machine's warranty, as many of them require you to use the manufacturer's cleaning solution to keep the warranty valid.

Alternative Options – Carpet Shampoo (For Machines)

Canada & USA

Biokleen	biokleenhome.com
Puracy	puracy.com

Carpet Stain Remover

This spot treatment should remove most fairly new stains that haven't had time to set yet. For very old stains that seem impossible to get out, try the Steam Iron trick on the next page.

Ingredients

- 1 cup (250 mL) warm water
- 2 tablespoons (30 mL) white vinegar
- 2 teaspoons (10 mL) Sal Suds (or clear dish soap)
- Baking soda
- Clean, absorbent towels/cloths (at least 2)

Directions

Mix the water, vinegar, and Sal Suds in a spray bottle and shake well. Sprinkle a thin layer of baking soda on the stain. Spray the cleaning solution to saturate the baking soda and let it fizz and bubble. Once the fizzing has stopped, start blotting the stain with the towel to soak up the solution. (For stubborn stains, you might need to gently rub the spot to loosen up the stain.)

Once you're done, rinse the area by pouring or sponging some cold water on the spot, and then blot with a clean towel. Continue to rinse the area until no more solution or stain comes up on the towel. To dry the area, just lay a thick towel over the spot and weigh it down with something heavy, like a pile of books.

Steam Iron Trick for Carpets

If you've tried the spot treatment method above without luck, you can try this nifty little trick I learned from a blog called creeklinehouse.com. You will use the same ingredients as the previous method, but this time you're going to utilize the magic power of an iron with a steam setting.

Ingredients

- ¾ cup (180 mL) water
- ¼ cup (60 mL) white vinegar
- 2–3 drops Sal Suds (or clear dish soap)
- Light-coloured washcloths
- An iron with a steam setting

Directions

Add the water, vinegar, and Sal Suds to a small bowl and stir to combine. Soak a washcloth in the solution, wring it out, and place it over the stain. Run your warm iron over the washcloth for a few seconds to steam the stain. Lift the cloth, and you should see the stain starting to transfer to the cloth. Keep placing a clean part of the cloth over the stain and steaming it until it's all removed from the carpet. Dry the area by laying down some dry towels.

Alternative Options – Carpet Stain Remover

Canada & USA

Better Life	cleanhappens.com
Biokleen Bac Out	biokleenhome.com
ECOS	ecos.com
Fit Organic	fitorganic.com
Greenshield Organic	greenshieldorganic.com
Nature Clean	natureclean.ca
Puracy	puracy.com

Africa

Earthsap	faithful-to-nature.co.za/earthsap

Floor Cleaner Guide

Use this guide to find the safest cleaner for your specific floor type. For the spray and wipe method, add the ingredients to a spray bottle, then spray directly on the floor and wipe with a damp cloth (either by hand or with a microfibre mop).

Laminate Floors

SPRAY & WIPE	MOP & BUCKET
• 1 cup (250 mL) distilled water • ½ cup (125 mL) white vinegar • ½ cup (125 mL) rubbing alcohol • 4–5 drops castile soap • 10–20 drops essential oils (optional; omit if you have pets)	It's not recommended to use a mop and bucket with laminate floors, since the excess water can warp the wood.

Tile Floors

Tile floors are best cleaned with a steam cleaner, or you can use the same recipe as laminate floors.

Bamboo Floors

Just a damp microfibre cloth or pad is all you need to clean bamboo and other unfinished hardwood floors. Wet the cloth or pad with water, squeeze out all the water and clean the floors by hand or with a microfibre mop.

Hardwood Floors

SPRAY & WIPE	MOP & BUCKET
• 2 cups (500 mL) water • 2 tablespoons (30 mL) white vinegar* • 5–10 drops essential oils (optional; omit if you have pets) *You can replace the vinegar with 1 teaspoon castile soap	• 1 gallon (4 litres) water • ½ cup (125 mL) white vinegar* • 10–20 drops essential oils (optional; omit if you have pets) *You can replace the vinegar with 1 teaspoon castile soap

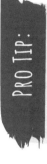

PRO TIP: Remove your shoes when you enter your home, and switch to indoor shoes or slippers if you like. The amount of dirt, bacteria, and impurities that are brought into your home just from your shoes is enough to make your skin crawl. BONUS: your floors will stay cleaner for longer, so it's a win-win!

Alternative Options – Floor Cleaners

Canada & USA

Aspen Clean	aspenclean.com
Attitude	attitudeliving.com
babyganics	babyganics.com
Better Life	cleanhappens.com
Biokleen	biokleenhome.com
Counter Culture	countercultureclean.com
Eco-Max	eco-max.com
Eco-Me	eco-me.com
ECOS	ecos.com
Planet Luxe	wellbeingisland.com
PUR Home (Black-owned; LW)	shoppurhome.com

Europe & UK

Elmkind (LW)	elmkind.co.uk
Greenscents	greenscents.co.uk
KINN	kinn-living.com
Ocean Saver (LW)	ocean-saver.com
Sodasan	sodasan.com
Sonett	sonett.eu

Australia & New Zealand

Abode	healthyhomeproducts.com.au
EcoLogic	martinandpleasance.com/brands/ecologic
EnviroCare Earth	envirocareearth.com.au
Euclove	euclove.com.au
Koala Eco	koala.eco
OurEco Clean	ourecoclean.com.au
Planet Luxe	wellbeingisland.com.au

Saba Organics	sabaorganics.com
Sonett	sonett.com.au
The Botanical Life Co.	thebotanicallifeco.com.au

Africa

Better Earth	betterearth.co.za
Earthsap	faithful-to-nature.co.za/earthsap
Mrs. Martin's	mrsmartins.co.za
Natural Orange	faithful-to-nature.co.za/natural-orange
So Pure	sopure.co.za

Asia

Gramp's	grampsasia.com
Pipper Standard	pippersingapore.com
Soapnut Republic	soapnutrepublic.com

Glass & Window Cleaner

Clean your windows and mirrors with this powerful combination that cuts through dirt and grease and leaves you with a streak-free shine.

Ingredients

- 2 cups (500 mL) warm water
- ¼ cup (60 mL) white vinegar
- ¼ cup (60 mL) rubbing alcohol
- 1 tablespoon (7 g) cornstarch

Directions

Add all the ingredients to a spray bottle and shake vigorously to combine. Spray on glass surfaces and wipe with a microfibre or cotton cloth. Buff to a shine with a dry microfibre cloth, if needed.

Alternative Options – Glass & Window Cleaner

Canada & USA

Aspen Clean	aspenclean.com
Attitude	attitudeliving.com
Better Life	cleanhappens.com
Biokleen	biokleenhome.com
Common Good (LW)	commongoodandco.com
Eco-Max	eco-max.com
ECOS	ecos.com
Ecostore	ecostoreusa.com
Greenshield Organic	greenshieldorganic.com
Koala Eco	koalaeco.com
Murchison-Hume	murchison-hume.com
Nature Clean	natureclean.ca
Pardo Naturals (Black-owned)	pardonaturals.com
Plant Therapy	planttherapy.com
PUR Home (Black-owned; LW)	shoppurhome.com
Saje Natural Wellness	saje.com

Europe & UK

Elmkind (LW)	elmkind.co.uk
Murchison-Hume	murchison-hume.ch
Ocean Saver (LW)	ocean-saver.com
Sonett	sonett.eu

Australia & New Zealand

Abode	healthyhomeproducts.com.au
Earthwise	earthwise.co.nz
EcoLogic	martinandpleasance.com/ brands/ecologic
Ecostore	ecostore.com.au
Euclove	euclove.com.au
Koala Eco	koala.eco
Murchison-Hume	murchison-hume.com.au
Planet Luxe	wellbeingisland.com.au
Saba Organics	sabaorganics.com
Simply Clean (LW)	simplyclean.com.au
Sonett	sonett.com.au
The Botanical Life Co.	thebotanicallifeco.com.au

Africa

Earthsap	faithful-to-nature.co.za/ earthsap
So Pure	sopure.co.za

Pest Control Spray

This simple spray works best to deter ants and spiders, but the peppermint oil is also effective against flies, beetles, and moths. Spray it around the perimeter of your home, near doorways and entry points, or wherever you see insects gathering.

Ingredients

- 2 cups (500 mL) distilled water
- 10 drops peppermint essential oil

Directions

Add all the ingredients to a spray bottle, and shake well to combine. Spray wherever you see insects gather, along doorways, cracks, and other entry points.

Alternately, you can soak cotton balls in peppermint oil and place them where you suspect insects are entering the home.

Warning

Do not use if you have pets in the house. If using the cotton ball suggestion, keep them out of reach of children.

Wood Furniture Polish

Keep your wood furniture gleaming with this simple polish that will remove grease, dirt, and fingerprints, and leave a glossy shine.

Ingredients

- ½ cup (125 mL) olive oil
- ¼ cup (60 mL) white vinegar
- 10–15 drops lemon essential oil (optional, degreases & adds scent)

Directions

Add all the ingredients to a spray bottle and shake well before each use. Make sure your surfaces are clean and dusted before using this polish. Lightly spray the solution on a clean towel or rag and polish surfaces. A little goes a long way!

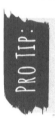

PRO TIP:

Keep dust, dander, and other allergens at bay by regularly dusting surfaces with a microfibre duster or cloth.

Alternative Options – Wood Furniture Polish

Canada & USA

Better Life	cleanhappens.com
Eco-Me	eco-me.com
ECOS	ecos.com
Pardo Naturals (Black-owned)	pardonaturals.com
Truce	truceclean.com

Europe & UK

Bio D	biod.co.uk
Greenscents	greenscents.co.uk

Australia & New Zealand

Oakwood	oakwoodproducts.com
OurEco Clean	ourecoclean.com.au

Africa

Wellness Warehouse	wellnesswarehouse.com

Asia

Esona	esonaonline.com

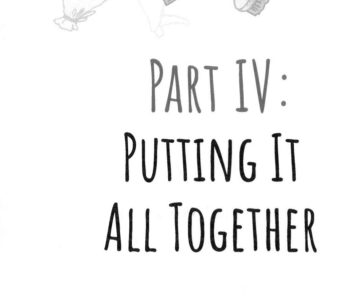

PART IV:
PUTTING IT
ALL TOGETHER

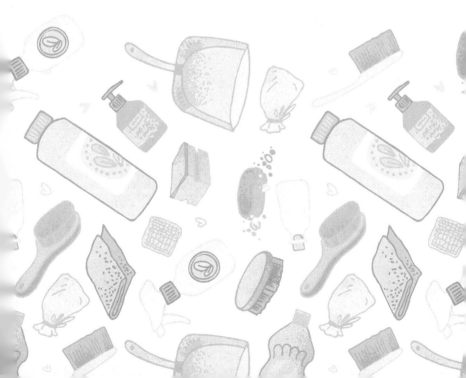

"

The hardest part is starting.
Once you get that out of the way,
you'll find the rest of the journey
much easier.

— SIMON SINEK

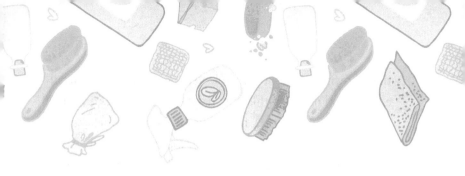

CHAPTER 15:
Taking the First Step

You just did something amazing. You read through this entire book and made it to the end—the finish line—so go ahead and do a little happy dance to celebrate!

You're well on your way to building your non-toxic home. You've laid the foundation, built the structural framework, and considered some of the ways you want to furnish and decorate that home with the safest products for your family.

Now comes the hard part—getting started. No matter what it is you're doing, starting is usually the most difficult part of any journey. It's much easier to complete a course on money management, for example, than it is to create a budget and pay off your debts. Signing up for a gym membership is simple enough. But showing up on that first day? Not so much.

Creating a non-toxic home is not much different. I can give you all the tools, resources, and information you need, but only you can take that first step to achieve your goal. Only you can make the first move. To help you do just that, I put together an Action Plan and a Quick Start Guide, which you can find on the following pages. A printable version of each is also available for you online at this link: naturesnurtureblog.com/book

The Action Plan is a fill-in-the-blank style worksheet to help you prioritize and map out your journey. Your Why Statement will be recorded, you will choose the first three products to replace in your home (although you'll still be focusing on one product at a time), and you will design a very specific plan of action. You'll create a mini road map using what you've learned from this book so that you can apply it to your journey.

The Quick Start Guide is what I refer to as "the foolproof plan." If you're still not sure where to begin, or if you're looking for the bare-bones minimum that you can do to get a real jump-start on your journey, this guide is for you! It includes a list of the easiest, most effective recipes you can make for each room. They're the ones I make and use most often in my own home, so they're quick wins to get you started.

With the Action Plan and the Quick Start Guide in your hands, you'll be able to start on the right foot and make great strides on your journey to a non-toxic home. But, again, it's on you to do the hard part and take that first step.

The Action Plan

Your Why Statement

Refer back to your "Why Statement" from Chapter 1. Write it down below:

....

....

Your Top Three Products

Fill in the chart below with the top three products you'd like to replace, whether you will make or buy them, and on what page they're listed in this book:

	PRODUCT	MAKE OR BUY?	PAGE #
1.			
2.			
3.			

Remember: you'll still only work through one product at a time. You're only listing your top three here so you can have a plan in place.

Action Plan continued on next page →

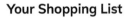

Your Shopping List

Keep a list of the ingredients you need to purchase to make your Top Three products. If you're going with a store-bought alternative, write the names of two or three brands you'd like to try.

PRODUCT 1	PRODUCT 2	PRODUCT 3

Download this Action Plan and other bonus content at:
naturesnurtureblog.com/book

Quick Start Guide

Here's a shortlist of the easiest, most effective recipes you can make for each room, along with their corresponding pages in this book:

Kitchen

All-Purpose Cleaner, p. 96
Scrubbing Powder, p. 122

Bathroom

All-Purpose Bathroom Cleaner, p. 129
Disinfectant Spray, p. 136
Foaming Hand Soap, p. 138
Toilet Bowl Cleaner, pp. 147-149

Laundry

Dryer Sheets, p. 162
Fabric Softener, p. 164

Living Areas

Carpet & Mattress Refresher, p. 190
Glass & Window Cleaner, p. 200

"

You may never know what results
come of your actions, but if
you do nothing, there will be
no results.

— Mahatma Gandhi

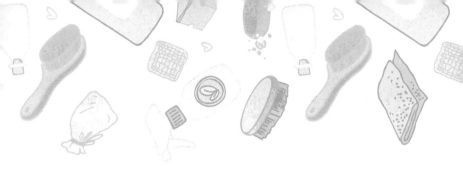

CHAPTER 16:
Forging Your Own Path

Our reasons for starting this journey—our *Whys*, if you will—may be different, but they share a common goal: we all want to live a better, healthier, more intentional life. Likewise, the routes you and I take to achieve our goals may look similar in many ways, but it's our personal circumstances that will dictate the little differences in our landscapes.

Our priorities, family dynamics, financial situations, physical and mental health—all of these will shape our journey and make it uniquely ours. But in the end, the destination is the same: a safe, healthy home environment for our families.

Remember that this will be a process. It's a marathon, not a sprint. You cannot create your non-toxic home overnight; it will take time and energy, but the results will speak for themselves. With that being said, here's my friendly disclaimer: do not put this off along with those *other* projects that you hope to get to someday. You know which ones I'm talking about. Writers call them "one-day novels"—as in "one day I'm going to write that novel." But of course, that auspicious day never comes.

There never seems to be enough time, enough energy, or enough money to get things going. Well, guess what? There will never be "enough." We are constantly working against time, trying to increase our energy levels, and figuring out how to save money in the process. If you delay this project, hoping to come back to it "one day," you and I both know the truth. It will slip deep down into the darkest recesses of your mind, never to be seen or heard from again.

Too dramatic? Perhaps. But how many one-day novels have you already let slip by the wayside? How many big ideas or grand plans have you gotten excited and inspired by, only to let them slowly wither away? And how many had you completely forgotten about until just now because I reminded you of them? Don't add yet another one to the pile. This one is too important, too valuable to allow it to fizzle out. This project has the potential to change the entire trajectory of your life—if you just start now.

Too many of us wait until a major tragedy strikes before making a big change in our lives. A serious medical diagnosis, a terrible accident, or the loss of a loved one can really shake us up and force us to reassess our priorities. And the things that we ignored for far too long suddenly shoot up to the top of our list in a matter of seconds.

But what if we were proactive about these matters? What if, before we were forced to see a doctor about a preventable illness, we instead took small steps today to take better care of our health? What if we could change our prognosis before it ever happened? How would that play out over the next 10, 20, or 30 years?

These are the kinds of questions that get me excited about this work. They're inherently hopeful and promising. That's the feeling I want to leave you with after you finish reading this book. I want you to know—to *believe*—that making small, incremental changes today can have a lasting impact on your life. The choices you make over the next few weeks will be the ones you thank yourself for in the coming years.

Maybe you've already started with other areas in your life— you're eating better, you're moving your body more, you're taking care of your mental health. That's awesome, and cleaning up your household products needs to be squarely on that list for a truly holistic health plan.

Armed with the knowledge and resources in this book, I'm confident you can live a more natural, non-toxic lifestyle, and finally take charge of your family's health. But you've got to put in the work. Read the labels, check those ingredients, and utilize the tools I've shared with you to get a head start.

Follow the roadmap that we explored in Chapter 9. The Small Steps Formula™ will become your best friend, so remember: one product at a time, before moving on to the next. Bookmark the specific products you want to switch out in the Room-by-Room Analysis. Fold down the page corners, add some sticky tabs, do whatever you need to save those pages. Then, together with your family, fill out your personalized Action Plan and hang it up somewhere that's easy to see.

Finally, and perhaps most importantly, always remember your *Why*. Let it guide you, let it steer you on your path, and let it be the means by which you carry on, regardless of the circumstances.

I wish you success and prosperity as you embark on your journey to a non-toxic home.

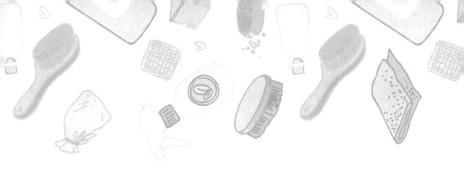

Acknowledgments

First and foremost, all praises and thanks are due to the Almighty, the One Most High, for the guidance, strength, and sustenance to complete this work. Alhamdulillah for everything.

This book would not be possible without the love and support of my husband, life partner, and best friend. Thank you, B, for always holding down the fort, for topping me up with endless cups of coffee, and for never making me feel guilty about retreating to my writing cave for days at a time. I'm so grateful to you.

To my readers and students throughout the years, thank you for continuously—and persistently—asking if I was ever going to write a book about this stuff. It's been a hot minute, but we did it, you guys! It's finally here!

A special shoutout to my small, but mighty, circle of friends, homegirls, and soulmates. I couldn't have asked for a more inspiring and encouraging group of women to have in my corner. To J, S, and N—you're my "ride or dies" in this life and until Jannah, insha'Allah.

I'm also indebted to my incredible team of editors, proof-readers, and designers, without whom this book would not be anywhere near as beautiful—or readable—as it is now. Thank you for putting up with my countless rounds of edits, additions, last-minute changes, and complete revamps. Your patience, diligence, and meticulous attention to the little details have turned my dream into a gorgeous reality. I truly appreciate you.

My family would probably disown me if I published a book and didn't thank them publicly, so dear family in all corners of the globe: thank you for loving me through thick and thin. Even (and especially) when I drove you crazy with all that "natural and non-toxic nonsense." Well, look who gets the last laugh!

And finally, the most important human in my life, the woman who made me who I am, despite all the odds: my mama. Thanks for always thinking more of me than I think of myself. You're my biggest cheerleader and my #1 fan. I love you.

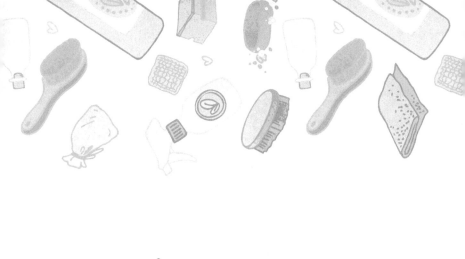

APPENDIX

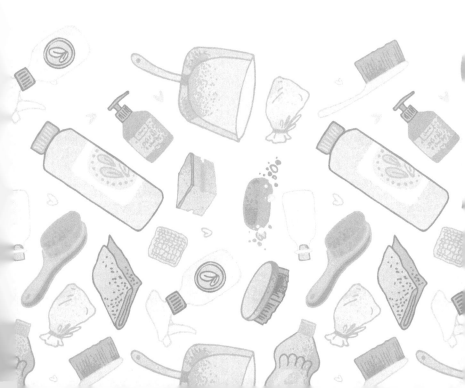

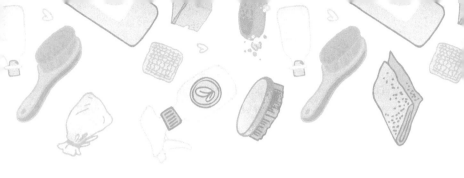

INGREDIENTS LIST

Below is a list of all the ingredients you'll need to make every cleaning recipe in this book. Most of them can be purchased locally at your supermarket; otherwise, they are readily available online.

Baking Soda	also called sodium bicarbonate or bicarb of soda; used in many recipes for scrubbing and freshening
Borax	also called sodium borate; this is NOT the same as boric acid; used in several dish, laundry, and bathroom recipes
Castile Soap	a natural vegetable-based soap, used in many recipes
Cornstarch	used in one recipe (glass cleaner) to remove spots
Citric Acid Powder	very effective at removing soap scum and hard water deposits; used in dish and laundry recipes

Distilled Water	boiled/cooled water is fine, but distilled is best for longer shelf life
Essential Oils	optional; provides nice scent and antimicrobial effects; avoid if you have pets
Hydrogen Peroxide	use standard 3% found at the pharmacy or chemist; excellent stain remover and disinfectant
Kosher Salt	also called coarse salt; used to thicken dish and laundry soap recipes for gel-like consistency
Lemons	great degreaser; can use lemon essential oil instead; only used in a few recipes
Olive Oil	only used in one recipe (wood polish)
Rubbing Alcohol	also called isopropyl alcohol or surgical spirits; used in many recipes to dry quickly and give streak-free shine
Sal Suds	a safe detergent from Dr. Bronner's brand; used mainly in dish and laundry recipes
Soap Flakes	or any natural bar soap, finely shredded; used in laundry recipes and liquid hand soap
Table Salt	a great abrasive and scrubbing agent
Vegetable Glycerin	gelling and thickening agent; only used in two recipes
Vinegar	white, distilled; used in many recipes
Washing Soda	also called soda ash; this is NOT the same as baking soda; used mostly in laundry recipes
Witch Hazel	only used in one recipe (air freshener) as a solvent
Xanthan Gum	gelling agent; used in just one toilet cleaning recipe

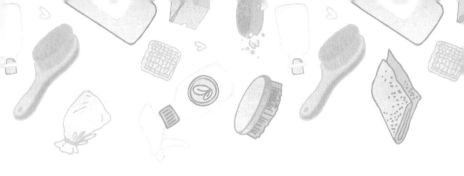

Equipment List

Along with the ingredients found on the previous page, you'll need a few pieces of equipment to make the recipes in this book. You might already have some of these at home, so feel free to upcycle them for your DIY cleaning kit. Just make sure to keep them separate from the ones you would use for food prep.

- ☐ Mixing bowl
- ☐ Measuring cups and spoons
- ☐ Kitchen scale
- ☐ Funnel
- ☐ Glass jars
- ☐ Spray bottles with a trigger nozzle
- ☐ Foaming pump bottles
- ☐ Cheese shaker or any container with holes in the lid
- ☐ Rubber gloves

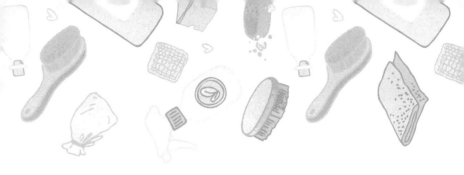

Supplies List

These are some cleaning supplies you might need in order to use the recipes you make from this book. They're not absolutely necessary, but they do make things much easier.

- ☐ Microfibre cloths
- ☐ Washcloths
- ☐ Sponges, preferably with a rough side
- ☐ Scrub brush
- ☐ Squeeze bottles
- ☐ Microfibre spray mop
- ☐ Large bucket

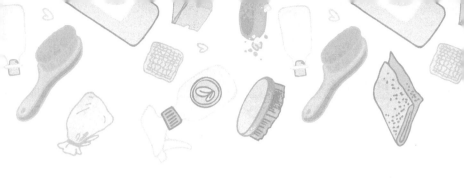

Where to Buy
Safer Products

I n recent years, with the increase in demand for safer products, many mainstream grocery stores have begun carrying more natural brands of cleaning products. This is great news! Several online retailers have also stepped up to offer a wide range of cleaning, health, and beauty products.

Online Shops

Canada & USA

Amazon Canada	amazon.ca
Amazon USA	amazon.com
Grove Collaborative	grove.co
Health Planet Canada	healthyplanetcanada.com
iHerb	iherb.com
Thrive Market	thrivemarket.com
Vita Save	vitasave.ca
Vitacost	vitacost.com
Well.ca	well.ca

Europe & UK

Amazon France	amazon.fr
Amazon Germany	amazon.de
Amazon Italy	amazon.it
Amazon Netherlands	amazon.nl
Amazon Spain	amazon.es
Amazon Sweden	amazon.se
Amazon UK	amazon.co.uk
Big Green Smile	biggreensmile.com
Ethical Superstore	ethicalsuperstore.com
iHerb	iherb.com
Natural Grocery	naturalgrocery.co.uk
Vitacost	vitacost.com

Australia & New Zealand

Amazon	amazon.com.au
Australian Organic Products	australianorganicproducts.com.au
Biome	biome.com.au
Buy Natural	buynatural.com.au
Flora and Fauna	floraandfauna.com.au
Hello Charlie	hellocharlie.com.au
iHerb	iherb.com
My Home & Co	myhomeandco.com.au
Natural Supply Co.	naturalsupplyco.com
Neatspiration	neatspiration.com.au
Nourished Life	nourishedlife.com.au
Organic Instinct	organicinstinct.net.au
Shop Naturally	shopnaturally.com.au
Vitacost	vitacost.com

Africa

Essentially Natural	essentiallynatural.co.za
Faithful to Nature	faithful-to-nature.co.za
iHerb	iherb.com
Organic Choice	organicchoice.co.za
Thrive	wethrive.co.za
Vitacost	vitacost.com
Wellness Warehouse	wellnesswarehouse.com

Asia

Amazon China	amazon.cn
Amazon India	amazon.in
Amazon Japan	amazon.co.jp
Amazon Singapore	amazon..sg
Amazon Turkey	amazon.com.tr
Amazon UAE	amazon.ae
Cold Storage	coldstorage.com.sg
Fair Price	fairprice.com.sg
iHerb	iherb.com
KBC	koreabeautycosmetics.com
Tulin	tulin.asia
Vitacost	vitacost.com

Latin America

Amazon Brazil	amazon.com.br
Amazon Mexico	amazon.com.mx
Denda	denda.com.mx | denda.cl
iHerb	iherb.com
Vitacost	vitacost.com

Middle East

Amazon	amazon.sa
Green JO	green-jo.com
Lulu	luluhypermarket.com
Ripe	ripeme.com
Tamimi	tamimimarkets.com

Physical Stores

Big Box Stores	*Target, Walmart, Costco, Aldi*
Grocery Stores and Supermarkets	*Publix, Kroger, Sainsbury's, Loblaw's, Tesco, Trader Joe's*
Health Food Stores	*Whole Foods, Healthy Planet, Goodness Me, Sprouts*
Local Food Co-Ops	
Pharmacies and Drug stores	*Walgreens, CVS, Shopper's*

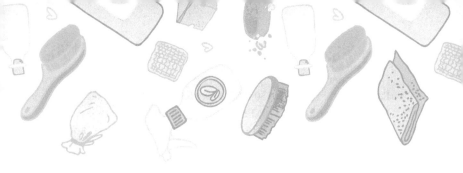

Directory of
Safer Products

Canada & USA

Europe & UK

Australia & New Zealand

Africa

Better Earth 99, 107, 109, 131, 151, 171, 184, 199
Cape of Storms 133, 173
Earthsap 99, 107, 109, 131, 133, 142, 151, 171, 173, 195, 199, 202
Enchantrix 99, 142, 151, 171
Mare & It is 99
Mrs. Martin's 99, 107, 142, 171, 184, 199
Natural Orange 99, 107, 133, 151, 173, 199
Nature Soap 99, 107, 142, 167, 173
Nu-Eco 99, 107, 113, 131, 142, 151, 167, 171, 184
Pro-Nature 146
Pure Simple (LW) 99, 107, 171, 178
So Pure 117, 137, 199, 202
The Apothecary 167
Triple Orange 107, 109
Wellness Warehouse 99, 109, 142, 171, 184, 205

Asia

Arau 107, 139, 167, 171
Bio-home 99, 107, 131, 171
Esona 99, 151, 171, 205
Ethique (LW) 99, 131, 178
Gramp's 99, 107, 178, 184, 199
Happy Elephant 109, 174
Miyoshi 107, 142, 171, 174, 178
Pax Naturon 107, 151, 171
Pipper Standard 99, 131, 139, 171, 178, 199
Soapnut Republic 99, 107, 133, 139, 151, 167, 171, 174, 199
Whamisa Organic Fruits 139

Latin America

Biogar 99, 171
Flor de Coco 99, 167, 174
Nama 171
Newen 99, 171
Pure & Sure 99

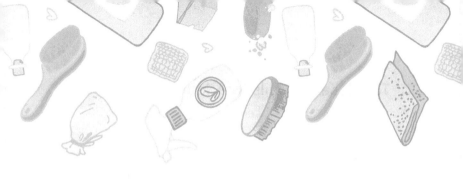

ESSENTIAL OILS FOR
CLEANING

E ssential oils are highly concentrated plant extracts. They are all natural and biodegradable, and many of them have powerful antibacterial, anti-fungal, and antiviral properties, making them very effective at cleaning your home.

With that said, I've purposely made them optional for most of the recipes in this book, because I don't want them to be the reason you don't try a recipe. If you do want to try using oils, make sure you're purchasing pure, undiluted oils. Below is a list of trusted brands I recommend, as well as the top essential oils to use in your cleaning products.

Essential Oil Brands

Aura Cacia	auracacia.com
Eden's Garden	edensgarden.com
Mountain Rose Herbs	mountainroseherbs.com
Plant Therapy	planttherapy.com
Rocky Mountain Oils	rockymountainoils.com
Saje Natural Wellness	saje.com

Top Essential Oils for Cleaning

Tea Tree & Thyme

Tea tree oil is the powerhouse of essential oils, as it is not only antiseptic and antimicrobial, it also kills fungus, insects, and most types of bacteria.[46] Thyme is also a very strong antibacterial oil and works as a great disinfectant.

Lemon & Orange

Both lemon and orange essential oils are great degreasers, making them an excellent choice for cleaning up around the stove and cooking areas. They also provide a bright, uplifting scent to your cleaning products. Citrus oils, in general, including lime oil, have also been found to be effective against several strands of bacteria, including *E coli*.[47]

Peppermint

Peppermint is a stimulant and is known for helping you focus, so it makes a great addition if you want to get some serious cleaning done. Beyond that, peppermint is a strong antiseptic and also makes a great bug repellant.

Lavender

Lavender not only promotes a sense of calm and relaxation, but it's also a mild disinfectant and antibacterial. This is a very common oil for giving your cleaners a nice, pleasant scent.

Cinnamon & Clove

Both cinnamon and clove oil can impart a warm, pleasing scent to your cleaning products. More importantly, they have shown significant antibacterial activity against several strands of bacteria, including *E. coli*.[48]

Essential Oil Safety

Essential oils are potent substances and should be handled with care. Yes, they come from natural plant sources; but as useful and effective as they are, they can also have serious consequences if not handled and used properly. Some basics to keep in mind:

Purity

Only purchase oils that are labeled "100% pure" to ensure they're not diluted with other substances. Shop around and compare prices; if the price is too good to be true, it probably is. The brands recommended above are a great place to start.

Pets

Some essential oils can be toxic to pets, so I would skip the essential oils in any cleaning products that may come into contact with your pet's skin/paws until you check with your veterinarian. Cats are especially sensitive since their livers are not able to metabolize certain compounds like those found in essential oils.

Children

Always keep essential oils out of reach of children.

You can find more detailed safety information, including individual profiles for each oil at usingeossafely.com.

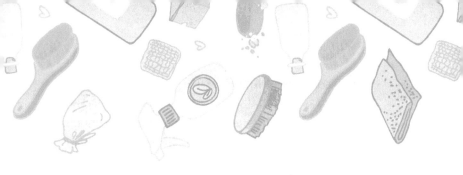

Safety Information

Although you're working with safer ingredients, you still need to exercise some caution with regards to how you handle them and how (or if) you can mix them. Just because two substances are safe on their own, doesn't mean they're safe (or effective) to mix.

Do Not Mix

- **Hydrogen Peroxide + Vinegar:** When combined, they create a corrosive product called peracetic acid, which can irritate skin, eyes, and lungs. You can apply one after the other to disinfect surfaces, but do not combine them in the same container.
- **Castile Soap + Vinegar:** When mixed in large quantities, they make un-saponified soap, which is a soap that has broken down into its original components. You end up with a curdled mess that is completely ineffective at cleaning.

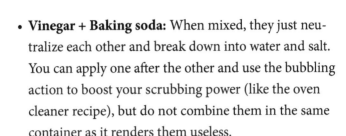

- **Vinegar + Baking soda:** When mixed, they just neutralize each other and break down into water and salt. You can apply one after the other and use the bubbling action to boost your scrubbing power (like the oven cleaner recipe), but do not combine them in the same container as it renders them useless.

Use Clean Tools

Make sure the tools, utensils, and containers you're using for your homemade products are properly cleaned beforehand. You don't want to introduce any bacteria or other contaminants into your products, rendering them ineffective, or worse, harmful for you and your family.

Label & Store

Just as you would with any products, make sure to properly label and store your cleaning products out of reach of children and pets. Again, just because you're using safer products, does not mean that they are safe to ingest!

Use Your Senses

If you ever notice an odd smell or a change in the texture of your DIY cleaning products, toss it and make a new batch. This is more likely to happen if you use tap water in your mixtures, as it has contaminants and minerals that can react with your products over time.

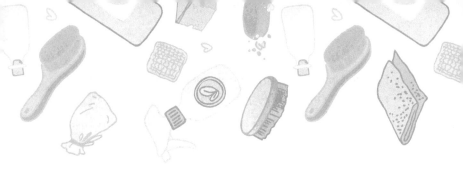

ADDITIONAL RESOURCES

Books

Creating a Healthy Household: The Ultimate Guide for Healthier, Safer, Less-Toxic Living (Bower, 2000)
Though a bit outdated, this detailed reference manual, written by someone who suffers from Multiple Chemical Sensitivities, discusses health concerns associated with indoor air pollution and provides alternatives for common household products.

Exposed: The Toxic Chemistry of Everyday Products and What's at Stake for American Power (Schapiro, 2009)
Written by an investigative journalist, this exposé uncovers the corporate and political powers that continue to allow dangerous chemicals into the U.S., all while being forced to provide much safer versions of those same products to the rest of the world.

How to Grow Fresh Air: 50 Houseplants that Purify Your Home and Office (Wolverton, 1996)

> Authored by the lead scientist of the 1989 NASA Clean Air Study, this book identifies houseplants that have been shown to remove toxins from indoor air. Each plant has its own profile page with photos, care instructions, and how effective it is at removing toxins.

Less Toxic Living: How to Reduce Your Everyday Exposure to Toxic Chemicals–an Introduction for Families (McCulloch, 2013)

> This book is well-researched and provides lots of information on dangerous chemicals in the home, as well as practical solutions.

Living in The Chemical Age: How an Ounce of Prevention Can Protect Your Family from a World of Toxins (Newman, Ph. D., 2018)

> A great guide that focuses specifically on contaminants in our food, water, personal care products, and pharmaceuticals, and how to avoid them if possible.

Naturally Clean: The Seventh Generation Guide to Safe & Healthy, Non-Toxic Cleaning (Hollender, Davis, et al., 2006)

> This book, from the leading brand of natural household products, explains the dangers of traditional cleaners and provides illuminating statistics that illustrate how the chemicals found in almost every home are known or likely to cause a host of serious health problems.

Our Stolen Future (Colburn, Dumanski, et al., 1997)
> An older book, but the information still rings true today, if not even more so. With a focus on how certain chemicals can interfere with our hormones and the health implications that come from that, this book poses the question: "what effects should health scientists be looking for" when determining the long-term health effects of exposure to these chemicals?"

Silent Spring (Carson, 2002)
> Dubbed "The classic that launched the environmental movement," this book was first published in 1962 and was the first to shed light on the indiscriminate use of pesticides, which led to massive, sweeping changes to the laws that affect our air, land, and water, effectively altering the course of history.

Your Body's Environmental Chemical Burden: A Resource Guide to Understanding and Avoiding Toxins (Klement, 2018)
> This resource guide references over 1500 published research papers that discuss the 25 most common chemicals in our homes, and how to limit our exposure to them.

Films

Antibiotic Resistance	(ABCTV Australia, 2016)
Blue Vinyl	(Gold & Helfand, 2002)
Chemerical: Redefining Clean for a New Generation	(Nisker, 2009)
Our Chemical Lives	(ABCTV Australia, 2015)
Overload: America's Toxic Love Story	(Eastman, 2019)
Plastic Planet	(Boote, 2009)
Stink!	(Whelan, 2015)
The Human Experiment	(Hardy & Nachman, 2013)
Trade Secrets	(PBS, 2001)
Unacceptable Levels	(Brown, 2013)

Websites

Campaign for Safe Cosmetics	safecosmetics.org
Consumer Product Information Database	whatsinproducts.com
Environmental Defence Canada	environmentaldefence.ca
Environmental Working Group	ewg.org
Good Guide	goodguide.com
Made Safe	madesafe.org
Nature's Nurture	naturesnurtureblog.com
Safer Chemicals, Healthy Families	saferchemicals.org
Silent Spring Institute	silentspring.org
Women's Voices for the Earth	womensvoices.org

Mobile Apps

CosmEthics (Europe)	This app lets you scan personal care and cosmetic products and analyzes their safety profile on the spot.
Detox Me	This clean lifestyle guide gives you simple tips for reducing your exposure to toxic chemicals.
EWG's Healthy Living	This app gives you the EWG ratings for over 130,000 personal care, cleaning, and food products.
Think Dirty	This mobile app lets you scan products, learn about their ingredients, and find safer options on the go.

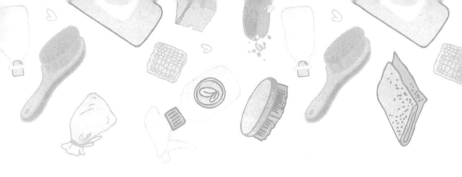

Endnotes

Chapter 1: Household Products and Our Health

[1] Government of Canada. (2019, August 22). *Volatile organic compounds.* https://canada.ca/en/health-canada/services/air-quality/indoor-air-contaminants/volatile-organic-compounds.html

[2] Government of Canada. (2019, August 22).

[3] United States Environmental Protection Agency. (2017, November 6). *Volatile organic compounds' impact on indoor air quality.* https://epa.gov/indoor-air-quality-iaq/volatile-organic-compounds-impact-indoor-air-quality

[4] United States Environmental Protection Agency. (2017, November 6).

[5] Xu, J., Szyszkowicz, M., Jovic, B., Cakmak, S., Austin, C.C., & Zhu, J. (2016). Estimation of indoor and outdoor ratios of selected volatile organic compounds in Canada. *Atmospheric Environment*, 141, 523-531. https://doi.org/10.1016/j.atmosenv.2016.07.031

[6] Gennings, C., Ellis, R., & Ritter, J. (2012). Linking empirical estimates of body burden of environmental chemicals and wellness using NHANES data. *Environment International*, 39(1), 56-65. https://doi.org/10.1016/j.envint.2011.09.002

Chapter 2: What is Hiding in Our Household Products?

[7] Maz, A. (2016, April 11). *Why companies don't show the ingredients in their cleaning products.* Upworthy. https://upworthy.com/why-companies-dont-show-the-ingredients-in-their-cleaning-products

8   Bickers, D. R., Calow, P., Greim, H. A., Hanifin, J.M., Rogers, A. E., Saurat, J., Sipes, I. G., Smith, R. L., & Tagami, H. (2003). The safety assessment of fragrance materials. *Regulatory Toxicology and Pharmacology*, 37(2), 218–273. https://doi.org/10.1016/S0273-2300(03)00003-5

Chapter 3: Safety Testing...or a Lack Thereof

9   Hollender, J., Davis, G., Hollender, M., & Doyle, R. (2006). *Naturally clean: The Seventh Generation guide to safe & healthy, non-toxic cleaning.* New Society Publishers. p. 53.

10 Vogel, S. A., & Roberts, J. A. (2011). Why the toxic substances control act needs an overhaul, and how to strengthen oversight of chemicals in the interim. *Environmental Challenges for Health*, 30(5). https://doi.org/10.1377/hlthaff.2011

11 Scialla, M. (2016, June 22). *It could take centuries for EPA to test all the unregulated chemicals under a new landmark bill.* PBS News Hour. https://www.pbs.org/newshour/science/it-could-take-centuries-for-epa-to-test-all-the-unregulated-chemicals-under-a-new-landmark-bill

12 Kollipara, P. (2015, March 19). *The bizarre way the U.S. regulates chemicals — letting them on the market first, then maybe studying them.* The Washington Post. https://washingtonpost.com/news/energy-environment/wp/2015/03/19/our-broken-congresss-latest-effort-to-fix-our-broken-toxic-chemicals-law

13 Kollipara, P. (2015, March 19).

14 Vogel, S. A., & Roberts, J. A. (2011).

15 EPA's Office of Pollution Prevention and Toxics. (1998, April). *Chemical hazard data availability study: What do we really know about the safety of high production volume chemicals?* https://noharm-uscanada.org/sites/default/files/documents-files/915/Chemical_Hazard_Data_Availability_Study_1998.pdf

16 Milman, O. (2019, May 22) *US cosmetics are full of chemicals banned by Europe – why?* The Guardian. https://theguardian.com/us-news/2019/may/22/chemicals-in-cosmetics-us-restricted-eu

17 Milman, O. (2019, May 22)

18 Government of Canada. (2018, January 8). *New substances program of the chemicals management plan.* https://www.canada.ca/en/health-canada/services/chemical-substances/chemicals-management-plan/initiatives/new-substances.html

19 Government of Canada. (2017, April 6). *The Canadian Environmental Protection Act, 1999 (CEPA 1999).* https://canada.ca/en/health-canada/services/chemical-substances/canada-approach-chemicals/canadian-environmental-protection-act-1999.html

[20] Burns, C. (2018, January 11). *'Natural' or 'organic' cosmetics? Don't trust marketing claims.* Environmental Working Group. https://www.ewg.org/news-and-analysis/2018/01/natural-or-organic-cosmetics-don-t-trust-marketing-claims

Chapter 5: The Worst Offenders

[21] Steinman, D., & Epstein, S. S. (1995). *The safe shopper's bible*, Macmillan. pp. 72–73.

[22] Rowdhwal, S. S., & Chen, J. (2018). Toxic effects of di-2-ethylhexyl phthalate: An overview. *BioMed Research International*, 2018. https://doi.org/10.1155/2018/1750368

[23] New Jersey Department of Health. (2011, July). *Hazardous substance fact sheet - Ammonium hydroxide.* https://nj.gov/health/eoh/rtkweb/documents/fs/0103.pdf

[24] Benzoni, T., & Hatcher, J. D. (2020, January). *Bleach toxicity.* StatPearls Publishing. https://ncbi.nlm.nih.gov/books/NBK441921

[25] National Toxicology Program, U.S. Department of Health and Human Services. (2016, November). *14th Report on Carcinogens – Ethylene Oxide.* https://ntp.niehs.nih.gov/ntp/roc/content/profiles/ethyleneoxide.pdf

[26] Campaign for Safe Cosmetics. (n.d.). *1,4-dioxane.* http://safecosmetics.org/get-the-facts/chemicals-of-concern/14-dioxane

[27] United States Environmental Protection Agency. (2017, November). *Technical fact sheet – 1,4-dioxane.* https://epa.gov/sites/production/files/2014-03/documents/ffrro_factsheet_contaminant_14-dioxane_january2014_final.pdf

[28] Keen, P.L., & Montforts, M. H. (2012). *Antimicrobial resistance in the environment.* John Wiley & Sons.

[29] Mount Sinai Selikoff Centers for Occupational Health. (n.d.). *Quaternary ammonium compounds in cleaning products: Health & safety information for health professionals.* https://med.nyu.edu/pophealth/sites/default/files/pophealth/QACs%20Info%20for%20Physicians_18.pdf

[30] Hollender, J., Davis, G., Hollender, M., & Doyle, R. (2006). *Naturally clean: The Seventh Generation guide to safe & healthy, non-toxic cleaning.* New Society Publishers. p. 59.

[31] U.S. Food & Drug Administration. (2019, May 16). *5 things to know about triclosan.* https://fda.gov/consumers/consumer-updates/5-things-know-about-triclosan

Chapter 6: What About the Germs?

[32] Ballantyne, C. (2007, June 7). *Strange but true: Antibacterial products may do more harm than good.* Scientific American. https://scientificamerican.com/article/strange-but-true-antibacterial-products-may-do-more-harm-than-good

[33] Roizen, M., & Oz, M. (2019, January 12). *Antibacterial soap, oversanitizing associated with allergies, autoimmune diseases: Drs. Oz and Roizen.* Cleveland.com. https://cleveland.com/healthfit/2012/09/antibacterial_soap_oversanitiz.html

[34] Zock, J. P., Plana, E., Jarvis, D., Antó, J. M., Kromhout, H., Kennedy, S. M., Künzli, N., Villani, S., Olivieri, M., Torén, K., Radon, K., Sunyer, J., Dahlman-Hoglund, A., Norbäck, D., & Kogevinas, M. (2007). The use of household cleaning sprays and adult asthma: an international longitudinal study. *American Journal of Respiratory and Critical Care Medicine*, 176(8), 735–741. https://doi.org/10.1164/rccm.200612-1793OC

[35] Michel, O. (2003). Role of lipopolysaccharide (LPS) in asthma and other pulmonary conditions. *Journal of Endotoxin Research*, 9(5), 293–300. https://doi.org/10.1177%2F09680519030090050401

[36] Centers for Disease Control and Prevention. (2020, November 27). *Coronavirus disease (COVID-19) – How to protect yourself & others.* https://www.cdc.gov/coronavirus/2019-ncov/prevent-getting-sick/prevention.html

[37] Prabuseenivasan, S., Jayakumar, M., & Ignacimuthu, S. (2006). In vitro antibacterial activity of some plant essential oils. *BMC Complementary and Alternative Medicine*, 6, 39. https://doi.org/10.1186/1472-6882-6-39

[38] Warnke, P. H., Lott, A. J. S., Sherry, E., Wiltfang, J., & Podschun, R. (2013, June). The ongoing battle against multi-resistant strains: In-vitro inhibition of hospital-acquired MRSA, VRE, Pseudomonas, ESBL E. coli and Klebsiella species in the presence of plant-derived antiseptic oils. *Journal of Cranio-Maxillofacial Surgery*, 41(4), 321-326. https://doi.org/10.1016/j.jcms.2012.10.012

Chapter 11: The Kitchen

[39] Rutala, W. A., Weber, D. J., the Healthcare Infection Control Practices Advisory Committee (HICPAC). (2019, May). *Guideline for Disinfection and Sterilization in Healthcare Facilities, 2008.* Centers for Disease Control and Prevention. https://www.cdc.gov/infectioncontrol/pdf/guidelines/disinfection-guidelines-H.pdf

[40] Fellman, B. (2009). The problem with plastics. *The Journal of the Yale School of Forestry & Environmental Studies*. http://environment.yale.edu/magazine/fall2009/the-problem-with-plastics

[41] Rutala, W. A., Weber, D. J., the Healthcare Infection Control Practices Advisory Committee (HICPAC). (2019, May). *Guideline for Disinfection and Sterilization in Healthcare Facilities, 2008.* Centers for Disease Control and Prevention. https://www.cdc.gov/infectioncontrol/pdf/guidelines/disinfection-guidelines-H.pdf

[42] Lester, S., Schade, M., & Weigand, C. (2008, June). *Volatile vinyl: The new shower curtain's chemical smell.* Center for Health, Environment and Justice. http://chej.org/wp-content/uploads/Volatile%20Vinyl%20-%20 REP%20008.pdf

Chapter 13: The Laundry Room

[43] UmmYusuf, S. (n.d.). *Your homemade laundry soap might be ruining your laundry.* Nature's Nurture. https://naturesnurtureblog.com/home-made-laundry-soap-problems

Chapter 14: The Living Areas

[44] Wolverton, B. C., Douglas, W. L., & Bounds, K. (1989, July 1). *A study of interior landscape plants for indoor air pollution abatement.* https:// archive.org/details/nasa_techdoc_19930072988/mode/2up

[45] American Society for the Prevention of Cruelty to Animals. (n.d.). *Poisonous plants: Toxic and non-toxic plants list.* https://aspca.org/pet-care/ animal-poison-control/toxic-and-non-toxic-plants

[46] Carson, C. F., Hammer, K. A., & Riley, T. V. (2006, January). Melaleuca alternifolia (Tea Tree) oil: A review of antimicrobial and other medicinal properties. *Clinical Microbiology Reviews*, 19(1), 50–62. https://doi.org/10.1128/CMR.19.1.50-62.2006

Appendix: Essential Oils for Cleaning

[47] Prabuseenivasan, S., Jayakumar, M., & Ignacimuthu, S. (2006). In vitro antibacterial activity of some plant essential oils. *BMC Complementary and Alternative Medicine*, 6, 39. https://doi.org/10.1186/1472-6882-6-39

[48] Prabuseenivasan, S., Jayakumar, M., & Ignacimuthu, S. (2006).

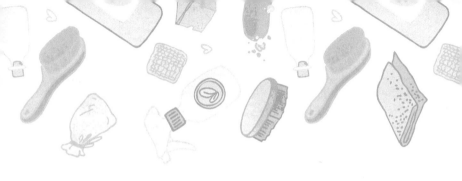

INDEX

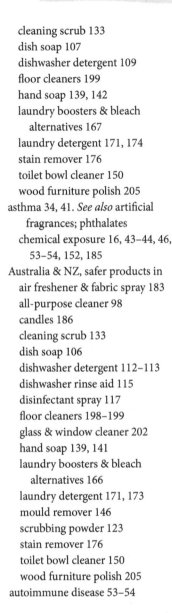

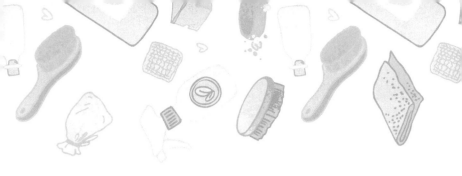

About the Author

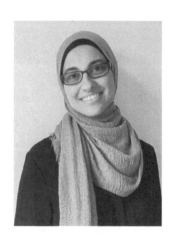

Sarah UmmYusuf is a writer and teacher who loves helping people take charge of their family's health. She created her blog, Nature's Nurture, in 2011 to document her journey to a non-toxic home, and has helped countless others start their own journeys. When she's not busy reading product labels or making her own cleaning products, you can find her chasing after her kiddos and drinking lots and lots of coffee. She lives in Toronto, Canada with her husband and three children.

Visit her blog at **naturesnurtureblog.com** and follow her on Instagram **@naturesnurture**

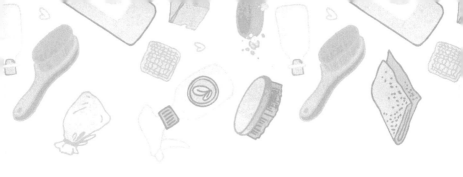

Level Up Your Journey!

We put together some amazing **Bonus Content** just for you! Visit **naturesnurtureblog.com/book** to access the complete library of bonus content that accompanies this book!

Here's what you'll get:

- Printable pages for the Action Plan, Quick Start Guide, Small Steps Formula, etc.
- Direct links for all resources in the book
- Recipe Cheat Sheets for each room in your home
- Printable Recipe Labels for your bottles and containers
- Checklists to mark off the products you will replace
- Reference Cards for the worst ingredients to avoid
- Printable quotes and artwork
- And much more!

naturesnurtureblog.com/book

Made in United States
Troutdale, OR
07/14/2024

21211495R00156